W9-AYR-509

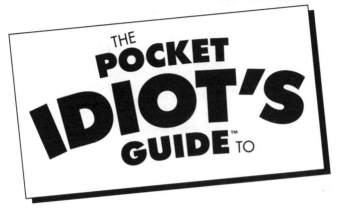

THE
POCKET
IDIOT'S
GUIDE TO

First Aid

*by Stephen J. Rosenberg, M.D.,
and Karla Dougherty*

alpha
books

A Division of Macmillan General Reference
1633 Broadway, 7th Floor, New York, NY 10019-6785

International Standard Book Number: 0-02-862015-1
Library of Congress Catalog Card Number: 97-073179

99   98   97   8   7   6   5   4   3

Interpretation of the printing code: the rightmost number of the first series of numbers is the year of the book's printing; the rightmost number of the second series of numbers is the number of the book's printing. For example, a printing code of 97-1 shows that the first printing occurred in 1997.

Printed in the United States of America

Publisher: Kathy Nebenhaus

Editor: Sora Song

Production Editor: Laura Uebelhor

Cover Designer: Mike Freeland

Illustrator: Judd Winick

Designer: Glenn Larsen

Indexer: Chris Barrick

Production Team: Tricia Flodder, Laure Robinson, Megan Wade

Contents

Introduction

First aid is one of those things you want to know how to perform but never have to use. None of us wants to think of someone being hurt or injured in a sudden accident. None of us wants to think of someone in pain. Unfortunately, life is filled with pain, along with its joys. And there are times when you need to know how to help ease painful situations.

When your child cuts herself, when your spouse hurts his head, when a toddler falls into deep water, or when bees spoil the family picnic, you need to use first aid skills. Those skills can make the difference between illness and health—and, sometimes, between life and death.

Learning first aid isn't a difficult task. The most important thing is to not be afraid. A cool head, good instincts, and step-by-step information are all you need.

That's where this book comes in. *The Pocket Idiot's Guide to First Aid* is the only sourcebook you'll ever need, if someone nearby gets hurt. This guide takes you from your medicine cabinet to first aid on the road. It provides a detailed description of everything from bruises to bandages, head injuries to heart attacks, smoke inhalation to sprains. And along the way, you'll find tidbits, interesting facts, insights, and vital tips that will make this book a must for every home and for every trip you take. Its small size makes it a handy little companion—tuck it away in a suitcase, in a glove compartment, or in the family medicine chest.

In the first couple of chapters, we'll take you through the real basics of first aid care. You'll learn exactly what to do when seconds count—without missing a beat. You'll know when to treat, why to treat, how to treat, and when it's best to wait for professional help. These "Principles" will be invaluable when you need to give first aid fast. You'll also get to peek inside the ideal medicine cabinet, and you'll find a detailed list of what you'll need for your own well-stocked "larder"—one that's always ready to tackle any emergency. We've also included some special tips, because not all families are the same. There are specific descriptions of things you'll need for children under 12, for teens, and for households with older adults.

The next 11 chapters are much more specific. In fact, they're the ones you'll most likely refer to again and again; they contain a complete lowdown of the most common situations that require first aid. Simply look up the accident or problem and follow the instructions for treating it.

How to Make This Book Work for You

Reading this book *before* an emergency arises will enable you to, as the scout motto says, "be prepared." But we've made this book accessible enough that you can refer to it any and every time an accident happens. And, just to make it even easier to use, we've added brief highlights at the beginning of each chapter to give you a "preview" of what's in store; this way you won't waste any time flipping through endless pages. After all, when seconds count, you want—and need—the information *now*.

Extras

No, we're not through yet. Just to ensure you've received a complete—and entertaining—education, we've added a series of shaded boxes throughout the book highlighting specific insights and precautions. You'll need these to understand thoroughly how to treat *any* first aid emergency:

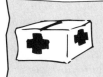

First Things First

This picture marks quick tips intended to facilitate first aid care and ensure safe treatment.

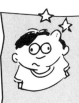

Ouch!

Look in boxes with this picture to find the important precautions you must take for a specific emergency. Read them. They can sometimes save a life!

First Aids

Boxes with this picture offer those definitions of medical words and descriptions you've always wanted to know but were, perhaps, too shy to ask. They'll make the injuries and their treatments more understandable and will provide you with razor-sharp instincts.

Special Thanks

The Pocket Idiot's Guide to First Aid would not have been possible without the patients who have received Dr. Rosenberg's care: the ones he saved and the ones for whom he did everything he could. A renowned expert in the field of neurology and geriatric emergencies, he knows, through experience and through his professorial lectures, from "whence he speaks."

Using his knowledge and expertise (and teaching abilities), he taught me (Karla Dougherty, the author of many books on medical subjects) the ins and outs of first aid care. He made me understand the nuances, watch the signals, and work fast under conditions that are not exactly calm.

We thank our editors, Sora Song and Laura Uebelhor, for their patience and expertise.

A special thank you also goes to our agent, Richard Parks, who has always stood by us during those "support needed" emergencies that, although not physical, are just as important to the creative mind.

Trademarks

All terms mentioned in this book that are known to be or are suspected of being trademarks or service marks have been appropriately capitalized. Alpha Books and Macmillan General Reference cannot attest to the accuracy of this information. Use of a term in this book should not be regarded as affecting the validity of any trademark or service mark.

One More Word(s) Before We Begin...

The 19th-century philosopher, Charles Edward Montague, once reported, "A gifted small girl has explained that pins are a great means of saving life, 'by not swallowing them.'" However, thanks to this complete, thorough, and easy-to-use first aid guide, if someone did happen to eat a handful of pins, you'd know exactly what to do.

Here's to health and successful first aid.

Need to Know Basics

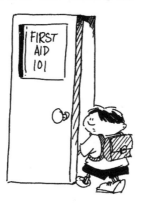

Boom! It happened. An accident. Maybe it happened on vacation. Maybe it was at the family picnic. Maybe it was on a quiet night during the week. Whatever the case, accidents do happen, and knowing at least the rudimentary rules of first aid can make a difference. You can help when seconds count.

Here you'll find the important basic principles you need to know to improve your reaction time, your efficiency, and your ability to handle emergency situations. With these basics under your belt, you can confidently rely on your instincts.

Principle 1: Use the Tools You Have

The words "first aid" probably conjure up visions of Band-Aids, ice compresses, and Ace bandages. In actuality, the most immediate and necessary tools for dealing with health emergencies aren't found in a kit or a cabinet. They are found on your person. They *are* your person—more specifically, your hands, your ears, your eyes, and your instincts.

Instincts are one thing, but don't underestimate the power of observation. When an experienced physician uses his or her gut to make a speedy diagnosis, it isn't just an instinctive feeling. To make a good, quick diagnosis, he also uses his eyes, ears, nose, and sense of touch. The clue is to know what to look for, and a good physician goes "right to the punch." Is the victim breathing? What does the breathing sound like? Are the eyes focused? Are there bruises and bumps on the body? What's the victim's reaction time when touched or spoken to? Combine your instincts with your powers of observation and you'll have an unbeatable combination to help save a life.

Principle 2: Don't Panic!

Easier said than done, right? If someone is unconscious, bleeding, crying, or hysterical, even the most composed "first aider" can panic.

Just remember: You'll be a much bigger help to the person in trouble if you remain calm and think through the situation. First, take a deep breath and count to three. Disassociate yourself from the crisis at hand. You can panic later—when trained help finally arrives.

Principle 3: Treat or Wait

It's often easy to see the injuries that need immediate attention. Using only your eyes and ears, you can usually identify and begin to treat profuse bleeding, respiratory distress, sprained arms and legs, and cardiac arrest. (See Chapter 2 for such key first aid treatments as making splints, making bandages, and performing mouth-to-mouth resuscitation.) But some conditions are not so obvious and require professional attention. Unconsciousness, for example, can be a sign of shock or head injury—both of which can be very serious. Unfortunately, these can't be treated with direct pressure or mouth-to-mouth. In fact, the best thing to do is cover the person with a blanket and get help fast.

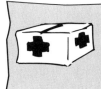

First Things First

Never move an unconscious person. If you aren't sure what's wrong, keep the injured party warm and still.

Principle 4: Know Emergency Numbers

It's a good feeling to be prepared. Whether you simply reach for your cellular, run half a block to the nearest phone, or pick up the extension in the kitchen, it's reassuring that you'll know exactly who to call. Every home should have an easily accessible list of emergency phone numbers that includes police, fire and ambulance, and poison control in addition to 911. If possible, program them into your phones for speed-dialing in an emergency.

Principle 5: Remember Your ABCs

Clearly, checking for vital signs is a priority in first aid care. That's why you'll hear us talk a lot about checking pulses, listening for breathing, and recognizing signs of shock. (Chapter 2 covers first aid treatment in the event of weak or no vital signs.)

To help you know which vital signs to check, remember your ABCs. These ABCs have nothing to do with reading and writing, but if you can think of them in the correct order, you *might* save a life.

➤ *Airways open.* Look: Be sure to see whether a person is breathing. Watch for steady intakes of breath and exhalations. Listen: Can you hear breathing? Is the breathing ragged or uneven? Help keep airways clear and accessible by placing one hand under an injured person's neck and gently tilting his or her head back to keep the mouth and nose unobstructed.

➤ *Breathing restored.* An unconscious person will breathe better if lying on his or her back. A conscious person will do better either sitting up or semireclining. Keep clothing around the neck and shoulders loose. Reassure the injured person, and keep him or her calm to eliminate the possibility of anxiety-induced conditions, such as hyperventilation.

If you detect shallow breathing or cannot detect any breathing, hook your fingers and check the person's throat to make sure nothing is clogging passageways. If the person doesn't appear to be breathing, perform mouth-to-mouth resuscitation (see Chapter 2). Get help as fast as you can.

➤ *Circulation maintained.* Checking for a pulse is as crucial as making sure the victim can breathe. The heart, after all, must send blood to the lungs, which pick up oxygen (and to the brain, which gives the command to breathe in the first place). Take the injured person's pulse (you'll learn how to in Chapter 2). If you can't find a pulse, begin CPR *if* you are trained and certified to do so. If not, perform mouth-to-mouth resuscitation (see Chapter 2) and scream for help.

Principle 6: Avoid Infection

In today's world, with ubiquitous threats of HIV (the virus that causes AIDS) and other infections, universal safety guidelines are always imperative. This principle pinpoints the necessary (and simple) precautions you'll need to take to protect yourself from contracting any infection or disease an injured person might have—and vice versa. Most deadly viruses are spread through an exchange of bodily fluids (blood, saliva, and even substances contained in vomit); the following universal guidelines are crucial for eliminating the risk of contact.

Wash Your Hands

Doctors "scrub up" before an operation for a reason. You won't have the luxury of a germ-free environment if you find yourself administering first aid in an emergency, but there are a few things you can do to protect the victim.

Wash your hands with hot water and soap, if possible. In case you're nowhere near a sink (or even a riverbed), cleanse your hands with a "wet nap"—a few of which you should keep in your first aid kit for just such a situation. If worse comes to worst, you can even use the alcohol or antibacterial lotion you'll be using to clean wounds.

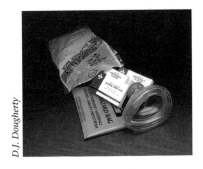

D.J. Dougherty

Universal safety devices prevent the spread of germs and infection.

Wear Gloves

It's a good idea to keep a couple pairs of disposable latex gloves in your first aid kit. When you're treating an open wound, gloves can protect you from most contagions. You can purchase latex gloves at hardware stores, medical supply stores, and some drugstores and supermarkets.

Wear a Gown, Apron, or Cover-Up

If you're in the midst of a life-or-death situation, you're probably not going to have those George Clooney-as-ER-doc protective greens at hand. But use common sense—especially if a person is bleeding and/or has an open wound. If you've been in the water, throw a cover-up over your swimsuit and bare skin, especially if you, too, have any vulnerable cuts or wounds. If you're wearing an open jacket, zip it up. Take precautions to keep you and the victim safe—unless seconds literally count.

Use Disposable Airway Bags

Airway bags let you perform mouth-to-mouth resuscitation without making contact with the other person's mouth. These handy gadgets can be found in many pre-packaged first aid kits today. Basically, an airway bag places a barrier between your mouth and the injured person's mouth to prevent the spread of disease.

Ouch!

When seconds count, there isn't always time to get an airway bag from your first aid kit (which might be in the car, parked 200 yards away). Although airway bags are best, you *can* perform mouth-to-mouth resuscitation safely without them. Use salt water, alcohol, or even soda poured on a cloth or a piece of clothing to wash the victim's mouth and nose. If the person is bleeding around the mouth or nose, use a handkerchief or other lightweight, porous cloth to keep the blood away from you as you work.

Use Protective Glasses and a Mask

Glasses or any type of goggles help protect your eyes from possible splashing from an open wound. If sunglasses are all you have available, you might be safer if you have them on—even if it's dark out.

Handkerchiefs make great masks. (Just ask any cowboy with a bandanna around his neck who's ever been caught in a dust storm.) To avoid possible airborne contagions, especially if you're helping a stranger whose medical history you don't know, simply tie a handkerchief or scarf around your mouth and nose. (Of course, you'll have to remove the mask to perform mouth-to-mouth resuscitation.)

Be Aware of Sharp Objects

If you have to treat a puncture wound caused by an arrow, knife, fishing hook, or rusty nail, apply antibacterial ointments and antiseptics around the wound. Never try to remove a large object; sometimes the only thing preventing profuse bleeding is the object in the hole. See Chapter 13 for specific instructions on when to remove a foreign object and when to leave it alone. And don't forget to wear your protective gear, just in case a puncture wound opens up further or the sharp object accidentally slashes you.

Principle 7: Know the Top 10

If time's a wastin', don't worry. Just follow the steps in this Top 10 list and you'll be prepared to begin your first aid care for real.

1. *Shout for help.* Don't be afraid to use your lungs and shout for help as soon as you begin first aid measures. Keep shouting for help until you know someone's heard you and taken action.

2. *Assess the situation and scout the territory.* If possible, ask the injured person what happened. Can she speak? Can she tell you how seriously she's been hurt? Also, look around and make sure that performing first aid isn't going to be hazardous to *your* health. Are there any exposed wires near the injured person? Are there toxic fumes or flames? In short, make sure you aren't in any danger before you start first aid—you won't be much help if you're injured, too.

3. *Determine whether the accident warrants a visit to a hospital—or simply a cleansing and a Band-Aid.* If the injured person can talk, great. If the person simply needs stitches, don't call for an ambulance, just make a trip to the emergency room. But if he or she is unconscious, you need to make that 911 call. Check those important ABCs: Are the airways clear? Is he or she breathing? What about circulation? Is there a pulse?

4. *If you are trained and certified in CPR and a person is choking or cannot breathe, begin CPR right away.* If you are not trained in CPR, do *not* attempt to resuscitate: You can break the ribs or puncture the lungs, and if the person is choking on something, you can actually force the object farther down his or her throat. If you don't know CPR, use mouth-to-mouth resuscitation techniques (see Chapter 2); for choking, use the Heimlich Maneuver (see Chapter 6).

Ouch!

Don't move an injured person if you don't have to. As long as you're not in a burning building or drowning at sea, it's best to let a person lie where he or she is. If the victim has back, head, or neck injuries, moving him or her can make the injuries worse or even cause permanent damage or death.

5. *Stop the bleeding.* If the injured person is bleeding, slow the flow by applying direct, even pressure with your hands and a cloth (see Chapter 2 for more details on how to stop bleeding). Remember to practice the universal guidelines for preventing infection. Lift up a bleeding limb if it doesn't cause substantial additional pain. Make and apply a tourniquet only as a last resort. (See Chapter 2 for details on using a tourniquet.)

6. *Treat any symptoms of shock.* If the victim is breathing harshly and is cold, clammy, nauseated, and pale, he or she might be in shock and could become unconscious at any time. (See Chapter 2 for treating shock.) If the victim is vomiting—also a sign of shock—you'll need to keep airways clear. Unless you suspect a back or neck injury, gently roll the victim's whole body to the side to keep airways open and prevent vomit from pooling in the back of the throat (which can cause choking). Cover the victim with a blanket if you see any signs of shock.

First Aids

CPR is short for cardiopulmonary resuscitation. When administered immediately to a patient suffering cardiac or respiratory distress, CPR can save the person's life. But you need to be certified in order to perform CPR correctly, so it's best to take a course to learn it. It's not safe to rely solely on what you've learned from reading a book.

7. *Look for a Medic Alert bracelet or necklace.* The Medic Alert identification tag (shown in the following figure) bears the name "Medic Alert" and displays the Greek symbol for medical care (a snake twisted around a staff). This bracelet provides medical and emergency personnel with life-sustaining information about the patient's medical history and special needs. The Medic Alert tag tells you whether the victim is diabetic, epileptic, or allergic to any medications—all of which can make a tremendous difference in the course of treatment. If there is no Medic Alert bracelet or necklace, check the injured person's wallet. Sometimes medical warnings are written on an ID card or driver's license.

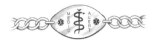

Look for a Medic Alert medallion like this on either a necklace or bracelet.

8. *Seek trained medical assistance.* At this point, if it's necessary, you can leave the injured person for a moment to summon help. In this world of cellular phones, it's nice to know we're only an arm's length away from 911. But what if neither you nor anyone around owns a portable phone? Shout for help or, as a last resort, run to the nearest pay phone. When you call for help, tell the police you want an ambulance with an EMT staff. Only trained personnel can help you with cardiac or respiratory problems, head traumas, poisoning, or fractures.

With or without medical alert information, you can make your call to 911 more efficient if you begin with your name, location, and the nature of the problem.

If you've performed steps 1 through 7, you can also inform them of additional things such as potential dangers in the locale (for example, toxic fumes, fire, or flooding) and whether the patient is breathing, bleeding, or appears to have broken bones. All of these things help the EMTs prepare themselves before they arrive on the scene.

 First Aids

EMT stands for Emergency Medical Technician. These are the trained medical technicians who arrive in a fully equipped ambulance, ready for any emergency and lifesaving technique. They get the victim to the hospital as quickly and as safely as possible.

9. *Never give an unconscious injured person anything by mouth.* This means no pills, no liquids—nothing.

Anything that must be taken orally can cause choking and difficulty breathing.

10. *Wait.* This is the hardest part of administering first aid care. When you've followed the steps above and done everything you can, all that's left is to wait for the ambulance to arrive. Unfortunately, minutes can feel like hours. While you're waiting, try to keep the injured person calm. You can provide comfort with a soothing voice or a gentle touch. "Sh. Don't worry. Help is almost here..." will help you cope as much as it will help the person you're treating.

Principle 8: The Complete First Aid Kit

Prepackaged first aid kits are great for the road. You can buy inexpensive, compact, "all-purpose" kits to stash in each of your cars and in almost every room of your house.

First Things First
The items in your first aid kit belong together and must be kept in one place. Remember to put back, or replace, any items you use.

Of course, space is not an issue when you're living at home. You have the luxury of filling your medicine cabinet with everything you might need—in the amounts you want. You can usually find all the items listed below in a drugstore or supermarket. If you don't want to keep them in a medicine cabinet, pack them into a childproof container and keep the container in a closet or kitchen cabinet—just make sure it's always easy to find and easy to reach. And needless to say, make sure everyone knows where it is. No matter what type of kit you have, you should place a list of emergency phone numbers inside the lid. Include numbers for your doctor, the local hospital, the poison control center, and more.

In order to have a useful first aid kit, you will need to purchase the following items; check them off as you put each one into your kit:

1. *Protective gear* to prevent the spread of infection. Remember those universal guidelines? Chances are, if an accident occurs within your home, you'll probably know the victim's medical background and might not have to bother with gloves, goggles, aprons, and dental dams (a device, similar to a football player's mouth gear, which protects your mouth from surprise fluid squirts). That said, it's always useful to have these items in your medicine cabinet just to be safe.   _____

2. *Adhesive bandages* in an assortment of sizes for any punctures, cuts, or minor scrapes. Be sure to buy individually wrapped, sterile bandages.   _____

3. *Sterile gauze pads*—also individually wrapped—may be useful for larger cuts, profuse bleeding, burns, and infections.   _____

4. *A roll of adhesive surgical tape* will come in handy when using gauze pads. You will need the tape to secure the cotton pad to the laceration. We recommend using *cloth* tape. It keeps a gauze bandage secured without the irritation or discomfort of the other adhesive tapes.   _____

5. *Scissors* may be necessary to cut tape, clothing, or bandages in emergency situations.

First Things First

Individualize your first aid kit to fit your family's needs. If someone is asthmatic, add an inhalator. If someone is allergic to bee stings, add an anaphylaxis (bee sting antidote) kit. If someone is diabetic, make sure you have insulin on hand.

---

6. *Elastic bandages,* or Ace bandages (the common brand name), may be used with clips for sprains and twists. _____

7. *Sterile cotton balls* are useful for applying ointments and antiseptics, and a *sterile cloth* is good for washing and dressing cuts and abrasions. _____

8. *Tweezers* come in handy for removing any foreign objects from a cut or for removing splinters. Although *needles* are usually good only for splinters, they can sometimes get small foreign objects out better. _____

9. *Matches* or a *childproof lighter* can be a useful addition to your medicine cabinet's first aid section. In an emergency, a flame will sterilize needles and tweezers. Just make sure you always keep matches and lighters out of the reach of tiny, curious hands. _____

10. *Rubbing alcohol* can be used to clean uten- _____
sils in your first aid kit, and it effectively
cleans cuts, scrapes, and minor wounds.
Antibacterial antiseptic lotions and ointments should be added to your homemade
kit as well. Bacitracin, Betadine, or Johnson
& Johnson's First Aid Cream are good all-
around antiseptics that will prevent infection on scraped knees, cuts, and wounds.
They also make excellent dressings without the sting of alcohol.

11. *Oral* and *rectal thermometers* are important _____
(and petroleum jelly for the rectal thermo-
meter). Fever can be a sign of shock,
poisoning, or infection.

12. *Calamine lotion,* which is used to relieve _____
itching and scratching, is great for insect
bites and hives. It also contains a healing
agent that's especially useful for poison ivy.

13. *Antihistamine tablets* are good to have _____
handy in case of an allergic reaction, an
attack of the sneezes and sniffles, a sinus
problem, or a migraine headache (all signs
of allergic reactions to pollen or dust). Benadryl is a good antihistamine, and it even
comes in a cream to treat superficial allergic
reactions, such as rashes and hives.

14. *Mineral oil* and *Q-tips* will do the job if you _____
need to remove ticks from the skin and
foreign objects from ears. Simply dab a little
oil on the Q-tip and gently touch the area
needing attention.

15. *Sterile eye wash* is a must for eye injuries. _____

16. *Syrup of ipecac* will induce vomiting in _____
case of poisoning. The sole purpose of
syrup of ipecac, which is made from a
South American root, is to trigger the
vomiting reflex. It's available in any drugstore and doesn't require a prescription to
purchase. Use syrup of ipecac only if you
know exactly what an injured person swallowed. Vomiting can worsen symptoms of
some poisons, such as petroleum and cor-
rosive chemical products. To be absolutely
certain whether to induce vomiting, call
your local poison center immediately.

17. *A bar of soap* or a container of antibac- _____
terial liquid soap should be ready to go
for cleaning wounds and washing your
hands. Sealed "wet naps" also work well.

18. *An ice pack* will reduce swelling, cool a _____
victim, and reduce fever. Many companies
now make "instant" ice packs that don't
need to be chilled (chemicals keep them
cold so you can store them in a first aid kit).

19. *A flashlight* comes in handy at home, in _____
case the power goes out. Be sure to check
the flashlight batteries frequently. You
should also keep *flares* in your car or boat
to alert passers-by of an emergency
condition. Flares not only prevent
unforeseen collisions in the dark, they
force other drivers to slow down (and
someone might just offer help or the
emergency phone call you desperately
need).

20. *Medicine for diarrhea,* such as Pepto-Bismol, _____
Imodium AD, or Mylanta, never seems to

be around when you need it. Make sure you keep some in your first aid kit.

21. *Aspirin, acetaminophen (Tylenol), and* _____
ibuprofen (Advil) tablets should all be on hand to relieve pain and reduce fever. Remember that some people are allergic to aspirin or have bleeding or stomach problems that aspirin can worsen. When in doubt, opt for the Tylenol or Advil. NEVER give aspirin for a fever to children under 18 years of age; they are particularly susceptible to Reye's Syndrome, a form of brain damage that can occur when aspirin is taken for a fever. Instead, give kids Tylenol for Children, or Pediaprofen (a child's version of ibuprofen). Ditto for pregnant moms.

22. *Large, triangular pieces of cloth (scarves)* will do _____
for makeshift slings, splints, and tourniquets.

Principle 9: For Children Under 12

Remember that trip your whole family took to Williamsburg—when your youngest child suddenly got the worst cold of her life? The fact is that young kids tend to experience sudden illnesses more often than their older siblings or parents. Further, young children need different doses of medication and treatment. They can take the same medications and ointments as their older counterparts, but NOT AS MUCH. In short, read the labels of your pain relievers, your cough syrups, and your creams before you use them for children. Even better, check out your drugstore shelf and pack a supply of baby aspirin and other specific children's medications in your first aid kit. Other special items for kids include:

1. *Baby aspirin*, but only for aches, pains, and strains. Kids under 18 years old with fevers should take Tylenol for Children or Pediaprofen (a child's version of Advil) to avoid the risk of Reye's Syndrome, a dangerous ailment that affects the nervous system.

2. *Warm blankets*.

3. *A small stuffed animal*.

4. *Towels* to use as makeshift pillows, immobilizing equipment for head and back injuries, or simply to wipe up dirt, sweat, and vomit.

5. *Baby powder* to add a soothing touch.

6. *Children's cough syrup*.

7. *A music box* or favorite cassette and Walkman for distraction.

8. *Adhesive tape* with "fun" designs and shapes.

9. *Cloth tape* (it's easier to remove).

10. *A bright bandanna* for use as a sling or splint (anything to help distract the child).

 First Things First
Children over 12 need special attention, too. First, make sure they don't panic. If soothing words don't help, calmly explain what you're doing and why. Have the teen become a part of your "first aid treatment team." It's a good distraction until help comes. Teens can handle most adult medications, but a few extra items that can help when a teenager is injured include a warm blanket, a pad and pencil in case he or she can't talk (and/or needs a distraction), a Walkman and a few favorite cassettes (also for distraction), and nonalcoholic cough medicine.

Principle 10: For Older Family Members

Here are some extras you might want to keep on hand specifically for adults (although they might come in handy for youngsters, too):

1. *Anaphylaxis kits* are essential if any family member is allergic to bee stings. This simple antidote will reduce inflammation and swelling in the airways and help the victim breathe again.

2. *Nitroglycerin tablets* are good to have on hand if anyone in your family has a history of heart pain or angina.

3. *Inhalators* are necessary for asthma sufferers. Keep several on hand in case it takes a while for help to arrive.

4. *Eye drops* soothe eyes irritated by an allergic reaction, and eye washes help flush out any chemicals that might have accidentally gotten in the eyes. (See Chapter 8 for specific eye first aid.)

5. *Ear drops* will help reduce earaches caused by infections and fevers. They will also help remove an overload of wax or a stubborn insect, and they can help restore inner ear equilibrium.

6. *A vial of glucose* isn't absolutely essential, but it comes in handy if someone feels a sudden drop in energy in the middle of the afternoon—it could be a low blood sugar reaction. The solution if you don't have any glucose? Keep a few packets of sugar in easy reach to place on the tongue.

7. *Insulin tablets* or *injections* are imperative in any first aid kit if someone you know has diabetes.

First Things First

Contrary to popular opinion, a "nip" of brandy is NOT good medicine. It doesn't keep you warm (in fact, alcohol lowers body temperature) or help you stay calm. That said, if you're the one performing the first aid, that brandy could taste mighty good after the crisis!

8. *A warm blanket* or one of those shiny, lightweight insulated covers (used by astronauts in space) will help keep your loved one warm.

9. *A plain brown paper "lunch bag"* can be used to ward off panic attacks. Simply have the victim breathe into a bag for several minutes to help steady his or her breathing. It's also a good idea to have a supply of anti-anxiety medication on hand if anyone in your family has a history of anxiety or panic attacks.

Chapter 2

When Emergencies Can't Wait: The Top 10 "How To"s

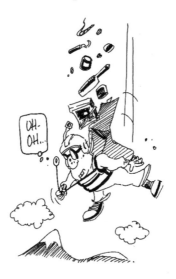

OH-
OH...

In This Chapter

➤ Taking a pulse and finding a heartbeat

➤ Stopping the bleeding and bandaging cuts

➤ Performing mouth-to-mouth resuscitation effectively

➤ Recognizing the signs of shock

➤ Keeping an injured person immobile

➤ Making an effective splint

Think of this chapter as a first aid map—one that will help you navigate the rules of performing basic first aid care. Here you'll find step-by-step instructions for taking a pulse. You'll also learn the basic procedures for treating a shock victim, and more. After reading this chapter, you'll be familiar with the 10 most necessary first aid skills.

"How To" #1: Taking a Pulse

There are several different ways to take a *pulse*. If you can't feel a pulse at one location, you'll need to try another area on the individual's body, as detailed in the following steps:

First Aids

The *pulse* is the rhythmic expanding and contracting of the arteries, caused by the blood moving through them. When the heart beats, the walls of the arteries swell with blood. Between beats, as the blood moves along, the walls shrink back to normal size. This regular swelling and shrinking is what you feel when you take a person's pulse.

1. Place your second (index) and third (middle) finger on the inside of the injured person's wrist. Your fingers should be right below the wrist crease and near the thumb (see the following figure). Press down.

Ouch!

Never use your thumb to take a pulse. It has a pulse of its own, so what you feel while trying to locate a pulse may be your own beating heart and not the injured person's.

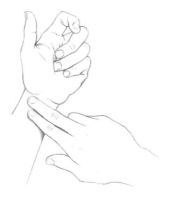

Take the pulse at the wrist.

2. If you can't feel a pulse at the wrist, try the carotid artery at the neck as shown in the next figure. This is located below the ear, on the side of the neck directly below the jaw. You should feel the artery as you exert pressure on the neck. (This is the best place to take a pulse if you have to give mouth-to-mouth resuscitation.)

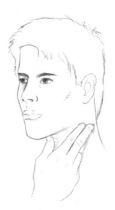

Take the pulse at the carotid artery.

3. If you still can't feel a pulse, try using the same two fingers on either side of the Adam's apple at the throat, the femoral pulse at the groin, or in between the muscles on the inner side of the upper arm.

4. As soon as you feel a pulse, count the pulse beats for 15 seconds (you'll need a watch), exerting pressure with your two fingers the whole time.

5. Multiply the number you get by four. This gives you the individual's total heartbeats per minute, or pulse rate.

A normal pulse ranges from 60 to 90 beats per minute. Babies can have pulse rates of up to 120 beats per minute; young children's pulses range from 80 to 160 beats per minute.

A rapid pulse can be a sign of shock or severe strain on the heart, such as an asthma attack or electrocution. If the beats are very faint or weak, an injured person might be in shock, his blood flow might be restricted, or he might be in a hypothermic condition (from the cold).

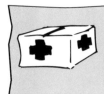

First Things First
If the pulse you find is very erratic, don't rely on math. Take a full 60 seconds to count the beats.

Practice taking a pulse on yourself or a family member so you'll be familiar with the process in case of an emergency.

"How To" #2: Listening to the Heartbeat
Listening to an injured person's heartbeat is just as important as taking his or her pulse. Obviously, a heartbeat

means the person is alive—even if the pulse is so weak that you can't feel it at any location. Here's how to listen to a heartbeat:

1. For men: Put your ear below the breastbone, slightly to the left of the left nipple.

   For women: Put your ear right below the left breast.

   For children: Put your ear slightly to the left of the left nipple.

2. Count the heartbeats you hear for one full minute.

A normal adult heart beats between 60 and 90 times per minute. Children and babies can have higher ranges. When a heartbeat is too fast, it can mean the victim is suffering from agitation or panic, shock, or fever. Treat each of those conditions as needed. (See the other "How to"s in this chapter.)

First Things First

To bring down a high fever, administer Tylenol or aspirin as directed on the bottle. Give the person a sitz bath: Fill a tub a quarter of the way with lukewarm water. Sponge the tepid water over the person to cool him or her off. Call your doctor!

"How To" #3: Stopping Bleeding

Where the bleeding is coming from is more important than the amount of blood you see. A minor cut can create profuse bleeding—as anyone who has cut him- or herself while shaving knows.

After you've determined where the cut is located, you can take appropriate steps to stop the bleeding, as described in the following paragraphs. And, as always, don't forget your universal safety measures.

Minor Scrapes

Treating minor cuts is relatively simple. If you have a child, you've most likely been doing it for years. You can tell a cut is minor if it's near the surface and isn't close to any important veins or arteries, which are near the heart, neck, thigh, and wrist.

That said, minor cuts can look a lot worse than they are. Here are some simple steps to follow when treating a minor cut:

1. After you've washed your hands, clean the wound with an antibacterial antiseptic and a clean sterile cloth. In an emergency where help and a first aid kit are nowhere in sight, a *clean* ripped T-shirt will do. Use an article of clothing only in absolute emergencies—clothes aren't always clean and may induce infection.

Ouch!
Don't use cotton balls to clean wounds. The tiny fibers might add to the injury. They can pull on scabs that might be forming, which can contaminate the wound below the surface.

2. Once you've applied a sterile cloth to cover the wound, apply direct pressure to the wound to slow the bleeding. Press firmly on the cut with your fingers and hand for several minutes without letting

up. (If the bleeding doesn't stop, the wound may be deeper than you thought. Get help as soon as possible.) After the wound stops bleeding, remove the pressure. Gently apply an antibiotic cream.

3. Cover the wound to avoid infection. Use adhesive bandages for small cuts and scrapes. Use nonstick gauze pads (taped down with adhesive tape) for large scrapes, surface area wounds, and wounds that are beginning to heal. Be careful when changing dressings because adhesives can pull on developing scabs.

4. If the bleeding continues, try elevating the limb slightly.

Deep Wounds

Treating and cleaning deep wounds must be left to medical professionals only; while waiting for help to arrive, however, you can still work to reduce bleeding. Apply pressure as described above in "Minor Scrapes." If the bleeding shows no sign of subsiding and continues to "gush" profusely, you might have to make a tourniquet. Tourniquets should be used only in life-or-death emergencies. Never use a tourniquet on the head, neck, or chest. Its unrelenting heavy pressure can stop the flow of oxygen to your heart, lungs, and brain—and cause permanent nerve and muscle damage. Tourniquets should only be used as a last resort for pulsing, spraying bleeding that cannot be controlled by direct pressure or elevating the limb. If you take a tourniquet off once you've put it on, bleeding could begin to flow twice as heavily as before. Always write down the time you applied the tourniquet and let the emergency squad know.

As a last resort only, follow these steps to make a tourniquet:

1. Find a scarf, a piece of cloth, or a sheet that is at least two inches wide. Wrap the material just above the wound three times.

2. Tie the ends in a tight half-knot.

3. Place a stick, a piece of wood, a pen, a utensil, or anything that is between five and ten inches long directly on the knot.

4. Tie the ends of the cloth around the stick item to the tourniquet with a double knot.

5. Twist the stick until the bleeding stops or at least decreases to a minor "trickle." Do not twist any further, as you might do more damage.

6. Keep the stick secure with another tourniquet knot or with another piece of cloth.

"How To" #4: Preventing Infection

Infection is a dangerous thing. Even after you've performed first aid measures exactly as described for cleaning wounds and stopping the bleeding from cuts, the victim is still not out of the woods. Infection can still set in, as much as hours or days after the injury.

In fact, infection is not just a problem with serious wounds. Minor wounds can also become infected, and they can become so seriously compromised that they lead to shock or coma. Signs of infection include:

➤ The area around the wound feels hot.

➤ The area around the wound is red.

➤ The injured person feels pain at the wound site.

➤ The wound site begins to swell.

➤ Fever.

➤ Chills.

To prevent severe infection and its fallout after the crisis is over, it's a good idea to change dressings on the wounds often and to check for signs of infection daily. If you notice any of the above symptoms of infection, treat them seriously. Call your doctor immediately.

"How To" #5: Performing Mouth-to-Mouth Resuscitation

If you've been certified and trained to do CPR, go to it at the first sign of breathing problems or an erratic heartbeat. If you don't know CPR, however, don't attempt it during your first emergency. Instead, get help immediately. While you're waiting, try mouth-to-mouth resuscitation; it can help save a life. The following figure shows an example of how you perform mouth-to-mouth; the following steps teach you how to do it:

1. First, ascertain whether the unconscious person is breathing at all. Bend down and place your ear near his or her mouth and nose and listen for sounds of respiration. Look at his or her chest and see whether it's rising and falling. Hopefully, all is not lost and the person is breathing, even faintly.

2. Position the injured person on his or her back.

3. Put on latex gloves for universal safety measures. Open his or her mouth and use your fingers to remove any obstructions in the throat or airway, as shown in the top portion of the figure.

4. To avoid transmission of deadly viruses via saliva, place your disposable airway bag over your mouth and over the injured person's mouth.

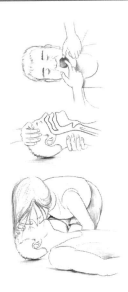

Performing mouth-to-mouth resuscitation.

5. Put one hand under the injured person's neck, and place the other hand on his or her forehead. Tilt the head back as far as you can to keep the airway clear. The injured person's mouth should be open. (See the middle portion of the figure.)

6. Pinch the nostrils to close them.

7. Take a deep breath.

8. Cover the injured person's mouth completely with your own. (See the bottom portion of the figure.)

9. Exhale hard four times into the injured person's mouth.

10. If you are working on an adult, pause for five seconds, then repeat steps 6 through 9, exhaling into the victim's mouth only once.

If you are working on a child or infant, pause for three seconds, then repeat steps 6 through 9, exhaling only once.

11. Repeat this exhaling process until the victim begins breathing, until you feel a pulse, or until help arrives. During the time you're not breathing into the person's mouth, continue to call for help.

12. Remember the ABCs you learned in Chapter 1. Use your brief pause between the resuscitations to check the victim's Airways, Breathing, and Circulation.

"How To" #6: Treating Shock

When an individual goes into shock, the body's chemistry goes out of whack. Balance must be restored—quickly. There are different degrees of shock, but expect some obvious symptoms whenever an accident occurs. Signs of shock include:

➤ Weakness

➤ Nausea

➤ Clammy, pale, cold skin

➤ Chills

➤ Erratic breathing

➤ Faintness or unconsciousness

➤ Weak and/or fast pulse

If a victim goes into shock, don't panic. Perform the ABCs of first aid: clear Airways, check Breathing, and maintain Circulation. Cover the injured person with a blanket to keep her warm. Then lay her down, keep her quiet, and elevate her feet to maximize blood flow to the brain.

Above all, get help as quickly as you can.

"How To" #7: Bandaging Wounds

Bandages have three purposes: to keep wounds clear of infection, to contain bleeding, and to provide additional protection and support. Sterile gauze is preferable, but in an emergency, just about anything will make a good bandage: scarves, T-shirts, socks, sheets, stockings, and even a belt.

Bandaging Head Wounds

If a wound affects the scalp, the bandage should be made by tying a kerchief on the head and knotting it in the back.

1. After putting on your protective gloves, stopping any bleeding, and cleaning the wound (see "How To" #3), fold a large bandanna-sized cloth into a triangle.

2. Place the bandage on the injured person's head, with the tip at the back.

3. Bring the two ends across the head, just above the ears, cross them in back, and bring the two ends back to the center of the forehead.

4. Tie the ends together.

5. Tuck the hem of the bandage snugly under the wrap.

If a wound only affects the forehead, put a square of sterile gauze pad over the wound. Then wrap a sterile gauze bandage around the head, "sweatband" style, as shown in the following figure. Circle the head at least three times to keep the dressing underneath in place. Cut and use adhesive tape to attach the ends, or tie them with a firm knot.

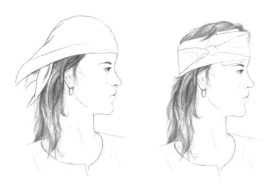

Bandages for large head wounds (left) and forehead wounds (right).

Ears and cheeks require a bandage that is more like an "old-fashioned toothache" style. These steps teach you how to apply such a bandage. The following figure illustrates the procedure.

1. Place a long, thick bandage under the chin.

2. Pull the ends up over the ears and cheeks, covering the treated wound.

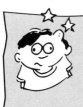

Ouch!
Do not use this "toothache"-style bandage if the injured person has a jaw problem or is vomiting. It can cause suffocation.

3. Cross the ends on one side, just above the ear.

4. Wrap the two ends in the opposite direction, making a "cross" by encircling the forehead and back of the head.

5. Tie the ends where the "cross" meets.

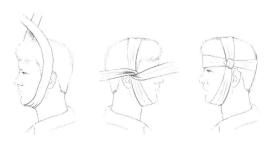

To bandage an ear or cheek wound, start by wrapping "tooth-ache" style. Then cross the ends on one side of the head and tie on the other side.

Wrapping Knee and Leg Wounds

To make a bandage that won't come apart on the knee or leg, follow these steps:

1. Clean and dress the wound while wearing protective gloves.

2. Bend the knee unless it causes pain. Then place the middle of your wide, long cloth at the underside of the knee joint (and over any dressing).

3. Wrap the cloth, in a spiral fashion, around the knee and the upper or lower leg (depending on the location of the wound). See the following figure for an example.

4. Bring the ends together. Tie them into a knot.

5. Secure the bandage with adhesive tape or safety pins.

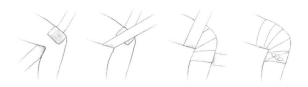

Wrap the knee.

Covering Arms and Elbows

Bandaging an arm or an elbow is very much like bandaging a knee or a leg. Once you've cleaned and dressed the wound with an antiseptic cream, follow these steps:

1. Bend the elbow you're wrapping.

2. Place the center of the cloth in the crook of the arm.

3. Spiral the two ends around the elbow and upper or lower arm (depending on the location of the wound). Then knot and tie the two ends.

Bandages for Wrists and Ankles

Think of an ice skater performing a figure-eight. That same twisting technique is effective for bandaging wrists and ankles. Here's how you wrap a wrist (after cleaning the wound):

1. Tape one end of a long, clean cloth or gauze roll to the palm of the injured hand.

2. Roll the gauze or cloth two or three times around the palm of the hand.

3. Bring the gauze or cloth across the palm of the hand and then in between the thumb and first finger (see the following figure).

4. Pull the gauze diagonally across the outside of the hand to the wrist.

5. Circle the wrist two or three times with the cloth, wrapping both the wrist and hand.

6. Repeat steps 1 through 5 until the wound and dressing are covered. Then secure the bandage at the wrist with adhesive tape or a safety pin.

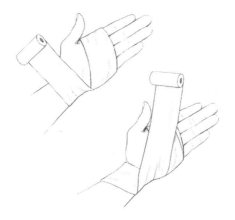

Wrap the bandage around the palm and then the wrist.

Follow these steps to use the same technique for wrapping an ankle:

1. Tape one end of a long, clean cloth or gauze roll to the instep of the injured person's foot.

2. Roll the gauze or cloth two or three times around the foot, moving from the instep to the back of foot, and from the back of foot to the instep.

3. Then bring the cloth up across the front of the foot and around the ankle (as shown in the next illustration).

4. Repeat this five to seven times, and then add one final circle around the ankle.

5. Secure at the ankle with adhesive tape or a safety pin.

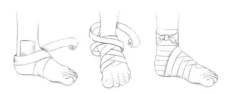

Bandage the instep and then the ankle.

Bandaging the Back and Neck

When someone suffers an injury to the back or neck, it's more important to keep him or her immobile than anything else. But sometimes that's not possible. Maybe the victim is face down in water and cannot breathe. Maybe he is vomiting and needs to have his head tilted. Maybe the person is bleeding profusely.

As is true of grammar, there are always exceptions to the rule. In those situations when bandaging a back or neck wound is necessary, move the injured person as little as possible. Keep bandages simple—just enough to stop the bleeding.

Wrapping Fingers and Toes

Bandaging wounded fingers or toes is just like bandaging any other part of the body but with smaller actions and smaller pieces of cloth. After you've put on protective gear and cleaned the wound, do the following:

1. Using a long roll of narrow gauze or a strip of cloth, place one end at the base of the finger or toe.

2. Hold the strip down with your thumb as you line the digit, by rolling the gauze up one side of the finger or toe and down the other side.

3. Continue lining the finger or toe—roll the gauze along the length of the digit, from one side of the finger or toe, over the top, down the other side, and back again. You'll have to hold the layers of gauze

down at both ends (at the base of the digit, on the front and back of the hand or foot), while you work.

4. After lining the finger or toe several layers thick, move the gauze roll to the side and begin to circle the finger or toe (you should now be moving the gauze perpendicular to the layers already lining the digit).

5. Knot the gauze at the base of the finger or toe as shown in the figure below.

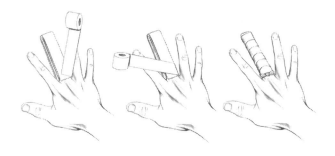

To bandage a finger or toe, first roll the gauze up and down, and then wrap the gauze around the digit. Finally, knot the bandage to complete the process.

A finger or toe bandage can also act as a splint in a pinch. Once you've bandaged the finger or toe (up and down, then in a spiral), pull the gauze roll down to the wrist or up to the ankle. Wrap around the wrist or ankle, and then pull back up and around the finger (or down and around the toe). Repeat several times and tie at the wrist or ankle. The following drawing illustrates how to wrap the hand in this way.

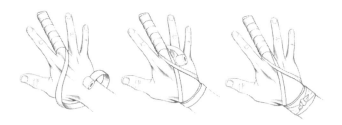

A finger or toe bandage can double as a splint.

"How To" #8: Immobilizing a Person with a Neck or Back Injury

The main reason you need to keep a person with a neck or back injury perfectly still is simple. Any movement, even the slightest bend or twist, can cause spinal cord damage, which in turn can result in permanent paralysis. Neck and back fractures do not necessarily mean spinal cord injury, but undue movement can create a problem that may not have been there before. The best position for an immobile person is flat on his or her back. But, if you find an injured person curled to the side or on the stomach, leave him or her in that position. Remember, there are very few reasons to move a person, especially if he or she is unconscious.

First Things First

Here's another exception to the "keeping an injured person immobile" rule. If someone is bleeding internally, it's important to roll him or her to the side to keep breathing passages open. Warning signs of internal bleeding include coughing up or vomiting blood, red or brown color in the urine, and red or black specks in the stool.

It's easy to tell someone to lie still, but what if he or she gets an itch or an unconscious twist? What if he or she contorts the body in pain? The best way to ensure immobility is to make a brace—almost all bulky items will do, but rolled-up towels, newspapers, blankets, and purses are especially good. Use heavy items to keep the lighter, bulky objects in place. These can include luggage, books, plants in heavy clay pots, and cinder blocks.

If an accident occurs in the middle of nowhere and if the injured victim is unconscious with possible back or neck injuries, you can still move him or her with a modicum of damage. Gently roll the individual onto a board and pull him or her to safety. If there's no board, use a blanket. And, if there aren't any blankets handy, gently pull the injured person by the arms or ankles.

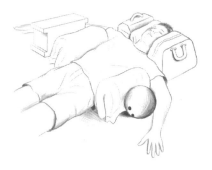

Use bulky and heavy items to immobilize an injured person.

"How To" #9: Making Slings and Splints

The "slings of outrageous fortune" might have created the emergency situation you find yourself in, but only a real, down-to-earth, and oh-so-practical sling will allow you to help someone with broken or bruised limbs. Here's an easy way to make an arm sling:

1. Fold a scarf or cloth into a triangle.

2. Put one corner of the triangle at the shoulder of the uninjured arm. Let the triangle dangle down the chest, the flat side closest to the uninjured arm.

3. For padding, place a pillow or newspaper, if available, on top of the cloth. Place the injured arm or bent elbow over the padding and the triangle dangling down the chest.

4. Pull the dangling corner of the triangle up around the neck to meet the corner at the shoulder of the uninjured arm. The injured arm should be inside the triangle, elbow covered as best as possible and fingers peeking out.

5. Tie the two corners together at the side of the neck—not at the back (you can damage the spine).

6. An ordinary safety pin will keep the sling in place. Using the safety pin, attach the point of the triangle at the elbow to the sling. (If you don't have a safety pin, twirl the point tightly until the arm is snug, then tuck the twirled point into the sling.)

7. Make sure the hand is four to five inches higher than the elbow to keep the blood flow circulating and to decrease pain. Adjust the sling, if necessary, by changing the knot at the neck.

When it comes to bones or joints, the most important first aid you can give is stabilization; keeping those bruised and broken bones immobile prevents further damage. Like bandages, splints provide support to broken bones, fractures, sprains, and painful joints, and they help immobilize them. If you don't have actual boards in your first aid kit, use your imagination. Almost any rigid, straight object will do. A rolled-up newspaper or magazine, a baseball bat, an umbrella, a broom handle, a folded blanket, or even a firm pillow may be used to provide stabilization. The following table contains suggestions for using basic, everyday items to create splints for various body parts.

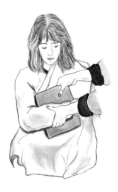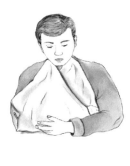

Making a sling.

Ouch!
Don't tie the splint too tight. It can cut off circulation. While waiting for help, continue to check the splint. Make sure that post-accident swelling isn't making the splint increasingly tight. Also, periodically take a pulse. If it becomes faint, loosen the splint.

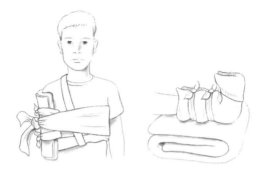

Use stiff items to create splints that immobilize joints.

Making Homemade Splints

Body Part	Splint Suggestion
Upper leg	Splint the two legs together.
Lower leg	Use a rolled-up newspaper, a baseball bat, or a broom handle.
Ankles and feet	A rolled-up newspaper or a magazine is best.
Back, upper torso, head, and neck	Only hard earth will do. Immobilize the person by placing folded blankets and pillows up against him or her and securing them with belts, ties, or sleeves. Remember not to move a person if a back or head injury is suspected.
Arms	An umbrella, a stout stick, a cane, a baseball bat—any of these will work.

continues

continued

Body Part	Splint Suggestion
Hands	A small board, a notebook, a picture frame, magazines, or newspapers will support a hand.
Fingers	Splint the problem finger with an adjacent finger.

"How To" #10: Preventing Panic

Trembling, crying, nausea, sweating, and mild gas pains are all typical reactions after an accident, especially if a person is in shock or terrible pain—don't be too concerned about such things. However, if these symptoms continue to worsen instead of passing, act fast. Panic builds upon itself, and it's contagious. What you don't need is a group of panicked people trying to administer first aid. Here are some techniques you can use to keep excess anxiety at bay:

➤ Talk in a low, soothing voice. Be consistent and repetitive—but confident—in your assurances. "Sh. You're not alone. I'm here. Help is on the way. Sh."

➤ Get the person to talk. A good distraction will keep his or her mind off the accident. Talk about, say, your vacation, the weather, or even the great watch he or she is wearing. If the victim is someone you don't know, try to get a name and address and a family contact. Listen and nod your head. You can even ask about his or her feelings—if he is scared or if he is in pain, for example—but don't scare him even more by letting your own emotions show. (Above all, don't yell.)

Chapter 3

Mother Nature's Bites, Stings, Scratches, and Rashes

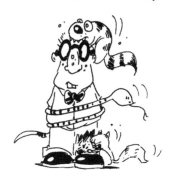

In This Chapter

➤ A rabid bite or a harmless nip?

➤ Jellyfish: Treating stings

➤ Insect bites: From spiders and bees to ticks and mosquitoes

➤ Irritating—and poisonous—plant life

We all love our animals, especially the pets that bring happiness to our families. But what about strange, rabid dogs and creepy, crawly insects? Or, what about those shiny, green leaves in the woods? This chapter will help you determine what to do when it comes to the bites, scratches, stings, and rashes created by "God's creatures," large and small.

Dog Bites and Cat Scratches et. al.

It might be true that household animals shouldn't "bite the hand that feeds them," but sometimes a pet dog or cat will lash out even at those they love—those who walk them, feed them, and hug them.

Stray animals, like raccoons, squirrels, and rats, are another matter. Obviously, they haven't been to the vet for their shots—and their bite can be considerably worse than their "bark." In order for an animal wound to qualify as a *bite,* it must break the skin. Whether you accidentally hit a dog's teeth or a cat scratches your skin, if the epidermis (skin) is broken, bacteria from the animal's saliva can seep into your open sore and result in infection. Animal bites can be very serious, so if a stray dog attacks someone on the street, or a rabid squirrel scratches an individual, first aid needs to be administered immediately. Use these steps to treat animal bites:

1. Stop any free-flowing, major bleeding (see Chapter 2). It can't wait.

2. Try to capture the animal before it gets away, or if it's someone's pet, get the name and address of the owner. Be careful not to be the pet's next victim. If the animal is wild, leave it alone. Do not attempt to capture it.

Ouch!
Do *not* use antibacterial lotion or cream on an animal bite. A bite is different from a cut or scrape; the bacteria in an animal's saliva can actually proliferate in certain creams.

3. Wash the wound for five full minutes (remember to wear gloves). Running water is preferable, but if supplies are limited, you can soak the affected area in still water; just make sure you change the water frequently. Washing the wound might cause bleeding again, but it's important to flush away any animal saliva completely.

4. Stop bleeding that might have occurred from washing the wound by adding direct pressure with a clean cloth. If possible, keep the injured area elevated above the heart until you get help. This will help control the bleeding. (See Chapter 2 for more details on how to stop bleeding.)

5. Bandage the wound with sterile gauze and see a doctor the same day.

6. If the injured person has not had a tetanus shot within the past eight years, make sure a physician administers the shot immediately. *Any* bite can make a person vulnerable to tetanus (otherwise known as "lockjaw").

The Danger Signs of Rabies

The only sure way to find out whether a warm-blooded critter has rabies is to perform laboratory tests. There are, however, certain signs that indicate the possibility of rabies. Keep an eye out for the following symptoms:

➤ The animal foams at the mouth, and its tongue hangs out.

➤ The animal can't seem to catch its breath; breathing is very labored.

➤ The animal suddenly lunges and snarls, ready to attack without provocation.

Another sign of rabies, especially in wild animals, is that the animal will approach and come near you instead of running away.

Rabies in its early stages is virtually undetectable, but some species are more prone to rabies than others. If an untagged dog, bat, raccoon, skunk, fox, rat, or squirrel comes close to you, it's best to walk away slowly so you don't anger or frighten the animal.

Avoiding Injury to Yourself

An old saying goes, "If you're not good to yourself, you can't be good to anyone else." If you get hurt by the same angry dog or nasty squirrel that hurt your companion, you won't be much help. Here are some bits of advice that might help you avoid this predicament:

➤ Blow a whistle or yell loudly—the animal should flee.

➤ If the person is not too badly bitten, carry or drag him or her to a safe place.

➤ This one's tough: Wait it out. As long as the animal is not continuing to attack, it's best to wait until it gets bored and leaves the scene completely.

➤ Try to disable the animal first. If you have no other recourse, if you are an expert marksman, and if you have a weapon available, you'll have to kill it. But make sure the brain is not damaged so it can be examined for rabies.

Jellyfish: A Water Menace

Ouch!

It's always a good idea to have a physician check out marine life bites, but not every bite is an emergency that requires *immediate* professional attention. Seek medical attention swiftly only if the victim is in shock; has a sting on the face (especially near the eyes or neck), which can cause dangerous swelling; or appears to be suffering a fever, swelling, or other atypical symptoms. Otherwise, if it's nothing more than a painful sting, a topical antibacterial ointment and dressing might suffice.

Jellyfish are aptly named—their gelatinous, cloudy bodies look like globs of jelly. But the unsightly body is not what's dangerous. The dangerous parts are actually the venom-filled cells that adhere to their dangling brownish tentacles; the poison is what causes pain when a jellyfish stings you.

Jellyfish "epidemics" are usually cyclical, occurring at specific times during the summer. One day, you'll be swimming in clear water; the next day, you'll find the ocean cloudy with jellyfish adrift in the waves. Avoid jellyfish altogether, but be aware that sometimes a long tentacle can get you even if the jellyfish body is far away.

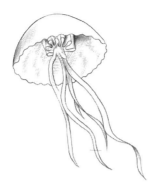

Jellyfish usually have a mushroom shape and a gel-like body.

Symptoms of a jellyfish sting can include:

➤ Immediate searing pain

➤ Swelling at the sight

➤ Red rash

➤ Nausea and vomiting

➤ Cramps

➤ Shock (in severe cases)

➤ Breathing problems (in severe cases)

If someone gets stung by a jellyfish, follow these steps to provide first aid for the wound:

1. Check vital signs. If the victim seems to be in shock or is having trouble breathing, immediately begin first aid for these conditions (see Chapter 2), and call for medical help.

2. Wrap your hand in a towel, or put on a protective glove, and wipe away any dangling tentacles from the wound site. (Be careful: You don't want the tentacles to touch your skin.)

3. Remove any jewelry near the site (even from the hand/wrist if the upper arm is stung).

4. Alcohol or ammonia will neutralize the poison. Simply wash the wound with either one. Alcohol can be used full strength, but you should dilute ammonia with fresh water (one part ammonia to four parts fresh water). Don't use salt water, which can dilute the ammonia's fighting power. If it's convenient, you can dilute a whole bottle of ammonia in two inches of bath water and have the victim sit in the bath for about an hour.

Ouch!

If you go to the beach, sand is a fact of life. It might be a nuisance when it sticks to your feet and clumps up in your swimsuit, but it also makes a great "towel" in an emergency. Sand won't cause an infection, and it will dry a wound when there's nothing else around.

5. Dry the wound site with sand, powder, or cornstarch. Don't apply creams or lotions before the sting is neutralized because such salves might trap the poison in the skin.

6. If there is swelling at the site, place a cold compress or an ice pack on the bite for 20 minutes every hour—or until help comes.

If the pain is very intense, try rinsing the bite site with some baking soda and water after you've followed your first aid steps. It can help decrease the pain until medical help arrives.

Even if the sting is mild and the victim feels fine soon after the episode, it's a good idea to keep watch for up to three days afterward. Jellyfish stings can get infected days after the incident. The best prevention? Antibacterial ointment —once the stinging sensation is gone. Before then…ouch!

First Aid for Creepy, Crawly Insects

A picnic can be ruined by a swarm of bees or a bustling army of ants. And a camping trip in the woods can send you home ridden with tick bites. As if getting bitten weren't bad enough itself, you could develop Lyme disease from an infected tick, or you could even fall fatally ill if you're allergic to certain insect bites. Read this section to learn everything about administering first aid.

At First Bite: Symptoms of Bee and Wasp Stings

One sting from a bee or a wasp will cause a burning feeling at the site of the bite. It will hurt—probably a lot—but the pain will be localized. The site will also probably swell, turn red, and itch. Multiple stings are more serious. They can cause fever, headache, muscle cramps, and drowsiness.

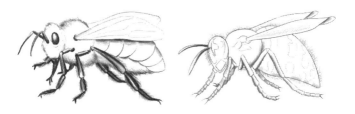

A honeybee (left) looks similar to a yellow jacket or hornet (right), but it's much less aggressive.

Stings aren't usually life threatening, but they can be if you have an allergy to the bee's venom. Signs of allergic reaction include nausea, excessive swelling, troubled breathing, bluish face and lips, choking, shock, and un-consciousness. If someone is sensitive to bee stings or if someone receives multiple stings (which can create an allergic reaction even in nonallergic persons), call for emergency help immediately. Watch the victim's vital signs and treat for shock or breathing difficulties if necessary (see Chapter 2).

Use the same treatment for bee stings (which leave venom sacs and stingers) and wasp stings (which leave stingers but no sacs).

1. If the stinger is clearly visible in the skin, gently "scoop" it out with the edge of a toothpick, a long fingernail, or a pocket knife (see the figure below).

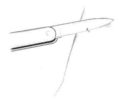

Use a knife to slide or scoop a stinger out.

2. Wash the affected area with soap and cold water. Then apply a cold compress or ice wrapped in a towel or cloth to alleviate pain and slow down the body's absorption of venom. (Always wrap the ice before placing it on the skin; plain ice sticks and causes more irritation.)

3. Apply calamine lotion or a mixture of baking soda and water to calm the inflammation and soothe the sting.

4. As long as the victim isn't allergic to aspirin, ibuprofen, or acetaminophen, you can give any one of them to him or her to help relieve the pain. If that seems to take care of it, the treatment is finished. If you are treating a more serious bee sting or multiple stings, continue to steps 5 through 8.

5. For multiple stings, soak the entire affected area in cool water. If necessary, place the victim in a tub of cool water. Add one tablespoon of baking soda for every quart of water.

6. If the victim has an allergic reaction, call for emergency help. Then have the victim lie in a prone position. Keep the affected area immobile and, if possible, lower than the heart. This will slow down the venom's circulation.

7. Tie a strip of cloth, a belt, a watchband, or the sleeve of a shirt two to four inches above the affected area. The bandage should be snug, but loose enough to fit a finger underneath it. (This ensures that you are not cutting off circulation completely.)

8. If the affected area starts to swell near the strip of cloth, tie another strip two to four inches above the first. Then remove the first strip.

Beware the Spider

Spiders—creepy, crawly critters that have been the stuff of nightmares, horror movies, Halloween decorations, and cries that would wake the dead ("Kill it, please. Aaaaack!"). Unfortunately, these arachnids (the name comes from Arachnida, the scientific name for the class to which spiders belong) get a bad rap. True, a few types are poisonous to humans and should be avoided at all costs. But garden-variety spiders, such as daddy longlegs, are usually harmless—and they even serve a good purpose on earth: They eat those pesky insects that attack our plants and flowers and invade our homes.

There are really only three types of spiders to worry about. Their bites can hurt and can contain poison. Bites from the spiders discussed below definitely require first aid treatment.

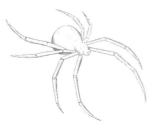

A black widow spider.

Black widow spiders, which are found mainly in the southwestern United States, are the queens of mean. These spiders measure only about ³/₄ inch in diameter and are recognizable by the red or yellow hourglass marking on the underside of their bellies. Symptoms of a black widow's bite may include an immediate sharp, severe pain; immediate redness at the site; profuse sweating; nausea and stomach cramps; difficulty breathing; and a tingling, burning feeling throughout the body.

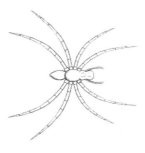

A brown recluse (violin) spider.

Brown recluse or **violin spiders** have small bodies with legs that look almost like strings. They are either yellow or tan and have a dark brown, fiddle-like design on their backs. They are quite small, measuring only $^1/_2$ inch to $^5/_8$ inch in size. Symptoms of brown recluse spider bites include severe pain occurring approximately eight hours after the bite, swelling at the bite site, blistering, chills and fever, aches and pains in the joints, nausea, and vomiting. Sometimes you can also see a kind of "target" around the bite—it might have a dusky or dark center and a red, raised, expanding edge.

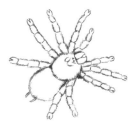

A tarantula.

Tarantulas really get a bad rap. These large, fuzzy spiders might look like rejected props from a B horror flick, but in reality, they're not so bad. You'll most likely find tarantulas in the southwestern United States and in South America. Tarantula bites occasionally cause intense pain at the bite site, but usually they only result in a bearable, short-term pain. Other possible symptoms include redness, swelling, a blistering and festered wound, numbness, difficulty breathing, nausea, and stomach cramps. Tarantula bites, however, are rarely fatal.

Treating Spider Bites

The treatment for spider bites is the same whether a person is bitten by a black widow, a brown recluse, or a tarantula. Follow these steps:

1. Seek medical help immediately: Dial 911 or drive to the doctor's office or the emergency room.

2. Have the victim lie down, and keep him or her quiet and warm.

3. Keep the bite area immobile and, if possible, lower than the heart (to slow the circulation of the venom).

4. Wash the bite site with soap and water.

5. If the person who was bitten is not allergic to acetaminophen, you can give him or her Tylenol to ease the pain. Be careful when dispensing pain relievers, though. In rare cases, aspirin can actually interfere with the blood's ability to clot and can "conspire" with the venom to facilitate the spread of poison. Your best bet is to give nothing, but if pain is severe, try Tylenol.

6. Tie a strip of cloth, a belt, a watchband, or the sleeve of a shirt two to four inches above the affected area. The bandage should be snug, but loose enough to fit a finger underneath it. (This ensures that you are not completely cutting off circulation.)

7. If the affected area starts to swell near the strip of cloth, tie another strip two to four inches above the first, and then remove the first strip.

8. Apply a cold compress or ice wrapped in a towel or cloth to alleviate the pain.

9. While you wait for help to arrive, observe the victim for signs of shock or breathing difficulties. (See Chapter 2 for symptoms of and treatment for those conditions.)

Treating Bites from Other Small, Annoying Critters

To treat the irritating bites from mosquitoes, bedbugs, chiggers, fleas, ants, and gnats, follow these steps:

1. Wash the bite site with soap and water.

2. Apply calamine lotion, a paste made of baking soda and water, or cold, wet cloths or compresses to relieve the itching.

3. Seek medical assistance if the person displays any of the following side effects:

   ➤ A fever within 10 days after the bite

   ➤ A throbbing pain that begins at the bite site within hours or even days

   ➤ Pus, redness, or swelling near the bite site

   ➤ Swollen glands

Any of these symptoms can signal a secondary infection. The person should see a medical professional in order to rule out serious diseases or allergies.

First Things First

If you squash or swat a mosquito away in the midst of the biting process, you'll actually experience more itching! Remnants of the mosquito's saliva are what cause itching, and if you let the mosquito finish sucking your blood, she'll remove much of her saliva along with your blood.

Tick Attack!

Ticks have received a lot of attention over the past several years. As transmitters of such deadly diseases as Rocky Mountain spotted fever and Lyme disease, ticks are considered Public Enemy Number One in the eyes of many.

Although Lyme disease has become a serious epidemic in certain parts of the country (specifically in the Rocky Mountains, in rural areas, and in northern climes), the truth is most ticks are harmless. The key is to make sure that you completely remove any tick that attaches itself to you.

Ouch!

Never pull, pinch, tear, or crush a tick that has already embedded itself in the skin. By doing so, you run the risk of removing only the body and not the head, which can lead to infection.

You'll definitely know a tick when you see one (at least when one attaches itself to you). They are tiny and oval in shape, and they have leathery black or dark brown skin. Unfortunately, they are not easily discernible when in their natural habitat: woods, trees, shrubs, deer, raccoons, and other forest creatures.

Instead of biting, ticks burrow. They dig into your skin head first and then hang out, contentedly sucking on your blood. If you see the tick when it's on the surface of the skin but has not yet burrowed, you can quickly pick it up with your fingers and crush it dead. If the tick has already embedded itself in your skin, however, getting it off of you can be somewhat tricky. Follow these steps to remove the tick:

1. Force the tick to "let go" by covering it completely with Vaseline, rubbing alcohol, or even salad oil or liquor. The oil closes off its breathing holes, and the tick should let go within 30 minutes.

2. Once the tick surrenders, pull it off the skin very carefully with tweezers.

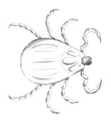

Ticks are usually harmless.

If you are at all fearful of accidentally leaving the head in the skin, go to a nearby walk-in or the emergency room for fast, efficient—and safe—removal.

If you wait the full 30 minutes and the tick refuses to surrender, proceed with these steps:

1. Using tweezers, turn the saturated tick counter-clockwise to make it release from the skin, making sure you pick up all its pieces. (It should come out fairly easily because of the oil.)

2. When the tick is out, wash the bite area thoroughly with soap and water.

3. Check for other ticks on the body and scalp.

Signs of Lyme Disease

The spread of Lyme disease has caused a certain amount of panic, especially among people who live in the Northeast. And statistics add to the scare: 50 percent of the deer ticks found in New Jersey carry Lyme disease, and raccoons, skunks, mice, and even solid earth itself can hold Lyme-carrying ticks.

First Aids

Lyme disease gets its name from the town of Lyme, Connecticut, where the first outbreak took place.

If you exhibit any of the following symptoms, see your physician as soon as possible. The presence of these symptoms doesn't necessarily mean that you have Lyme disease, but they can indicate other types of infection that might need medical attention.

➤ Swelling of the joints

➤ Swollen glands

➤ Fever within 10 days

➤ Throbbing pain at the bite site

➤ Pus oozing from the site

➤ Severe headaches

➤ A red, ring-like rash at the bite site within a month

➤ Chronic fatigue

If Lyme disease is not treated within the first few months, it can infect the heart or nervous system. It can also cause chronic arthritis. If you think you might have been bitten by a tick carrying Lyme disease, don't hesitate to have a blood test or contact your doctor. It's simple, it's easy, and it will put your mind at ease.

First Things First

Preventing tick bites is a matter of common sense. Wear long-sleeved shirts, long pants, caps, socks, and shoes when hiking in the woods or vacationing in areas that might be tick-infested. Choose light-colored clothing so that ticks will be more visible on you. Also, use insect repellent and spray your campsite with insecticides. And at the end of the day, you should always inspect your skin for ticks.

Poison I-I-I-IVY, Poison I-I-IVEE

Like the old song says, some of the worst skin rashes come from plants and trees. Poison ivy, poison oak, and poison sumac all produce an oily substance that can irritate most people's skin.

➤ **Poison ivy** is a green plant that grows low to the ground. It always appears as a shiny cluster of three reddish-green, teardrop-shaped leaves.

➤ **Poison oak** looks a lot like grape ivy. It's a vine with clusters of three leaves, sometimes three clusters to a branch. All the leaves have wavy edges.

➤ **Poison sumac** is usually found on trees in forests, but it can also grow on a bush. Its leaves are pointed like a palm frond and grow in pairs, except at the tip where there is always one leaf.

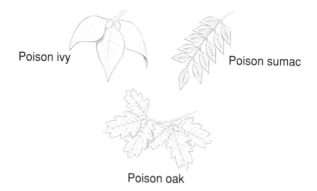

Poison ivy

Poison sumac

Poison oak

Poison ivy, poison oak, and poison sumac can cause severe rashes and itching.

Symptoms of the irritation caused by the three poison plants include red rashes (sometimes accompanied by small blisters), itching, headache, and fever. Coming into contact with these plants, however, is rarely fatal. (In fact, it doesn't require professional help—unless a person suffers a severe allergic reaction.) To prevent symptoms from spreading, follow these steps:

Ouch!

If someone happens to eat poison ivy, poison oak, or poison sumac, he or she should seek medical attention immediately. It can cause shock or breathing problems. (See Chapter 2 for treatment of such conditions.)

1. Take off any clothes that have come into contact with the poisonous plant and wash them in hot water.

2. Wash any part of the skin (especially where a rash appears) that might have come in contact with contaminated clothes or the plant itself. Use soap and hot water.

3. Wipe the skin with a cotton ball, a tissue, or a washcloth dipped in alcohol.

4. Apply calamine lotion to relieve discomfort and itching.

Chapter 4

Breathing Lessons

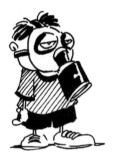

In This Chapter

➤ Handling breathing problems when seconds count

➤ Helping an asthma victim stay calm and comfortable

➤ Treating hyperventilation

➤ Dealing with an allergy attack

It's a frightening feeling when you can't catch your breath. Breathing problems are particularly scary because they can be their own worst enemy: Difficulty breathing creates anxiety, which makes the breathing problem even worse.

If someone around you is having problems breathing, it's important that *you* stay calm. Practice the principles of first aid care that you learned in Chapter 1: Don't panic, call for help, check the pulse, and place the injured person in a position that's best for him or her to breathe and to keep airways clear. (Most likely, the best position to ease breathing is either sitting up or semireclining.)

Breathing problems range from hyperventilation to asthma to allergy attacks, each of which has its own first aid treatment. These conditions can be tricky—sometimes they appear to be worse than they actually are, and other times they really are as serious as they look—so you have to be on your toes if you want to help. Your best bet is to read through this chapter and get a better feel for what to do when a breathing crisis occurs.

Helping the Asthma Sufferer to Breathe

When someone suddenly can't catch his or her breath, it's hard to stay cool. But that's exactly when calm, sound logic can mean the difference between life and death. *Asthma* is a common ailment; millions of Americans suffer its breathless slings. In many cases, someone having an asthma attack will know what to do. He or she may have an inhaler (a tube-like apparatus that you place in the mouth and pump with your hand) handy, which can aid breathing until help arrives.

But what if it's a child who suddenly can't catch his or her breath? Or a colleague or a stranger who doesn't have an inhaler at hand?

The first step is to recognize an asthma attack for what it is: It's not simply a case of hyperventilation, which occurs when a person literally breathes in too much oxygen and begins feeling dizzy and anxious, has chest pains, and feels tingling in the fingers and toes. An asthma attack sounds terrible; a person is literally fighting to catch his or her breath. He might lean over, move around, or act quite agitated, or he might sit in a chair with his head back using all his body's energy to breathe. There might be a cough, a rasping of breath, or a rattle. Breathing itself will use almost the whole upper torso, the neck, the shoulders, and, of course, the mouth.

First Aids

Acute asthma is associated with shortness of breath accompanied by wheezing. During an attack, the bronchial tubes constrict, impairing the flow of air into the lungs.

If any of these signs occur, try to get help as fast as you can. If the person has an inhalator, use it. Although you cannot be sure an asthma attack is in progress, the longer you wait for help, the more serious the attack will become. Remember, asthma can kill if it's not treated early enough. If you wait too long, even an inhalator won't help.

The main goal before help comes is to get the person to breathe as normally as possible. This is done through position, comfort, and relaxation.

➤ *Position:* Have the victim sit up or lean back in a semireclining position, whichever is the most comfortable. Do *not* let the person lie flat; it can make breathing even more difficult. Use an inhalator if the person has one or if you have one available.

➤ *Comfort:* Loosen any clothing around the neck and chest.

➤ *Relaxation:* Say soothing words and use calm motions to keep anxiety at bay.

Helping During Hyperventilation

First Things First

Because it's difficult to distinguish between hyperventilation and asthma, find out if the person having difficulty has any history of anxiety disorder or asthma. If you can't get an answer, it's better to be safe than sorry. Perform first aid for asthma, making sure the injured person is comfortable and his or her clothes are loosened, before trying hyperventilation techniques.

Although its root might be anxiety, the sensations that accompany hyperventilation are very real. The sufferer may experience the sense of not catching one's breath, the feeling of overwhelming terror that something is wrong, and the feeling that there is a loss of control. Hyperventilation can mimic an asthma attack or a heart condition. It occurs during an acute anxiety attack. Symptoms can include:

➤ Numbness in the hands, feet, and mouth

➤ A tingling sensation in the fingers or toes

➤ Overwhelming feelings of panic

➤ Chest pain

➤ Light-headedness

➤ Inability to catch one's breath

Although these symptoms are very real, they are not the source of the problem. Overbreathing is the cause: A person actually breathes in too much oxygen.

To stop hyperventilation in its tracks, simply use a paper bag as described here:

1. Have the hyperventilating person breathe slowly into a paper bag that's held closely around his or her mouth and nose.

2. The person should breathe like this for five to seven minutes.

3. Talk to the individual the entire time. Try to distract the person and make him or her feel comfortable and safe.

4. If symptoms fail to improve or the person loses consciousness, take him or her to the emergency room.

First Things First

If you don't have a paper bag, plain old hands will do. Simply have the person cup his or her hands over the mouth and nose and breathe in and out for at least five minutes.

That's all it should take. When the person breathes back in the carbon dioxide that he or she just exhaled, the correct chemical balance in the blood is restored and the physical symptoms cease.

When a person hyperventilates, emergency medical assistance is usually not necessary, as long as the procedures above are followed. But try to see a physician just in case; what looks like hyperventilation could be the onset of asthma or a severe allergic reaction that requires medication for relief.

Breathing Difficulties from Allergies

Parents often refer to this condition as *croup*. Health professionals call it allergies. These allergies affect the bronchial and respiratory systems. Rather than causing hives or itchy, red skin, allergies that affect breathing cause the throat to swell, constricting the airway and making it difficult to inhale.

First Aids

Croup is a "reactive airway syndrome." A virus (or other infection) causes the airway to become hyperactive and overly sensitive to stimuli. This results in spasms in the airway and wheezing. Once the inflammation dies down (which can take several weeks), the airway returns to normal. Antihistamines used to treat hay fever and allergies aren't always effective in treating croup; these medications are designed to combat conditions that affect the entire bronchial system, not just the airway (as in croup).

Symptoms of this type of breathing problem include wheezing, hoarseness, and a harsh cough. To administer first aid for such symptoms, follow these steps:

1. Call for medical assistance.

2. If a shower is nearby, create a "steam room" by turning the hot water on high with the shower curtain closed. If the person is an adult, hold him upright so that the steam is focused on his face.

   If the affected person is a child, lift her on your shoulders and have her breathe in the steamed air. (Be careful not to let any of the hot water splash on either one of you.)

3. Use your own judgment when it comes to steam. It can't hurt, but it might not be of any benefit either. If the steam helps restore breathing, keep the patient inside for up to 10 minutes, but never leave him or her unattended. Keep a vigil.

Ouch!
If the sufferer is drooling or is having difficulty swallowing along with difficulty breathing, go to the emergency room immediately. These symptoms are typical of epiglotitis, which can look like croup but can be fatal. Children are especially vulnerable.

4. After the person having difficulty leaves the "steam room," have him or her lie down, head slightly elevated. Towel the person dry and cover him or her with a warm blanket.

5. If the breathing problems begin anew, put him or her back in the steam. Continue the process until help arrives.

Sometimes the previous steps are all you need to clear breathing passageways. If the victim is starting to breathe easier and you are at home and have access to a vaporizer, place it close to the person's bed. A good night's sleep might do the trick.

Dealing with Dangerous Allergies

Sometimes allergic reactions can be more serious than asthma attacks, and seconds really count. A bee sting, an allergy to seafood or some other food (such as peanuts), or an allergy to certain weeds or flowers may be dangerous. Any of these can create an anaphylactic reaction, in which the throat swells so much that a person eventually won't be able to breathe at all. In this situation, the only recourse is to:

1. Call an ambulance.

2. Make the victim as comfortable as possible.

3. Follow the first aid instructions for asthma and allergies, above.

An epinephrine medication must be administered to neutralize the allergic reaction. People who have anaphylactic-reaction allergies are usually aware of their symptoms. They sometimes carry epinephrine injection kits prescribed by their doctors for anaphylactic emergencies. A person who has this allergy is usually trained in giving the injection. But if the victim is incapacitated, you will have to do it.

If a person stops breathing before help arrives, mouth-to-mouth resuscitation is your only course of action (see Chapter 2). Remember that breathing has stopped because of inflammation, congested airways, or a "deluge" of immune-resistant chemicals. Therefore, medication that decreases the inflammation and the harmful chemicals is the only thing that will work. Try an inhalator if the emergency becomes acute.

Don't forget to look for a Medic Alert bracelet. These bracelets can contain vital information that could ease allergic reactions and even save lives.

Chapter 5

Things That Go Bump (and Burn and Shock) in the Night

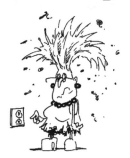

Bumps and bruises are the most common type of injury, and in most cases they require the least amount of first aid. Electric shocks, on the other hand, are much more dangerous; some of the worst shocks come from common household items and outlets. If you don't know the correct first aid procedures, you can actually make bumps, bruises, burns, and electric shocks worse. You can even hurt yourself in the interim.

In this chapter, we'll go from the least serious to the most serious injuries, showing you first aid treatment step-by-step all the way.

Scrapes, Cuts, Bumps, and Bruises

Bumps and bruises are damage that occurs in the soft tissue under the skin. If a person suffers a cut, scrape, bump, or bruise and meets the following conditions, there is no need to call for medical assistance:

➤ The injury is small (less than $1/2$ inch around).

➤ There is no bleeding, or only slight bleeding. Make sure you follow universal safety guidelines, such as wearing protective gloves, to prevent the spread of HIV and other dangerous infections. (See Chapter 2 for first aid care for bleeding.)

➤ The victim is not in excessive pain.

➤ The victim does not feel numbness or tingling.

➤ The victim is not suffering any paralysis.

Ouch!
If the injury swells noticeably, the bump could signal a bone or joint injury. And, if too many bruises start appearing too quickly, it could signal a serious circulatory problem.

➤ The victim does not seem to have any broken bones or dislocation at the joints. (If the victim is in a great amount of pain and the shoulder, leg, arm, or ankle appears to be lying or hanging at an awkward angle, there is a good chance he or she has a broken bone or a dislocated joint.)

Cut and Scrape First Aid

Here are simple first aid procedures for treating minor scrapes and cuts:

1. Wash a skin scrape or minor cut with mild soap and lukewarm water.

2. Apply Bacitracin or some other type of antibacterial cream or spray to prevent infection.

3. Cover the wound with a Band-Aid or a sterile gauze pad secured with tape.

Serious Bruises, Bumps, and Swelling First Aid

A cut and a bruise, with or without swelling, are basically the same thing, except that one occurs *at* the body's surface while the other occurs *under* the surface, in the soft tissue below the skin. In fact, the ugly black and blue marks you see when you bruise are really blood clots that form under the skin. The worse they look, the more they are clotting and healing.

Because bruises (and their potential partner, swelling) don't break through the skin, they require a different first aid treatment than do minor cuts and scrapes. Follow these steps for treating bruises:

1. Immediately apply an ice pack to the bruise to re- duce swelling. (If an ice pack isn't available, use ice wrapped in a cloth or as cold a compress as you can make.)

2. If possible, elevate the bruised area so that it's higher than the heart. This keeps blood from "pooling" in the affected area (and thus creating more internal bleeding and swelling).

3. Keep the bruise elevated for approximately 15 minutes if the wound is minor. If the bruise is severe and covers a large portion of the body, call for help. (See Chapter 2 for immobilizing techniques, if necessary; see Chapter 11 for information on treating sprains and breaks.) Keep a severe bruise elevated for at least an hour or until a trained emergency care team arrives.

First Aids

A *blister* is a built-up, fluid-filled irritation under the surface of the skin. A *blood blister* is a red blister that contains blood. A *fever blister* is another name for a cold sore or a herpes simplex at the lips. None of these are dangerous, but if they are accompanied by excessive pain or fever or if they grow larger, you should see your physician for proper drainage and possible medication. Don't pop them yourself—you run the risk of infection.

4. If the bruise doesn't appear to be getting any better and more than 24 hours have passed, see your physician.

5. Seek prompt medical help if there is any swelling around the bruise, especially if it occurs at a joint. This can signal danger to nerves, muscles, and bones, all of which require a trained physician's attention.

The Warning Signs of Internal Bleeding

A slight amount of bleeding that creates a bruise under the skin is one thing, but hemorrhaging is quite another. Internal bleeding can be serious and can affect a person's vital organs. The symptoms of internal bleeding are similar to those of shock:

➤ Pale, clammy skin

➤ Chills

➤ Cold hands and feet

➤ Dilated pupils

➤ Rapid, weak pulse

➤ Major swelling at the injury site

➤ Major or immediate black and blue marks at the wound

First Aids

Hemorrhaging is another word for uncontrollable bleeding. Because it's caused by breakage in blood vessel walls, it's usually internal, which means you can't always tell when a person is bleeding to death.

Unfortunately, first aid procedures will not stop internal bleeding. The best thing to do is to call for help immediately. Then proceed with the first aid steps for shock (see Chapter 2).

First Aid for Burns

Burns are unsightly, frightening, and very painful. But they can be treated with simple first aid steps. In fact, they are the one injury that *must* be treated before medical help arrives. Unless they're treated right away, burns will keep getting worse—they'll sink deeper below the surface of the skin because the heat continues to do damage.

First Aids

When it comes to burns, *degree* has nothing to do with temperature. The terms first-degree, second-degree, and third-degree identify the severity of a burn. First-degree is the least harmful, and third-degree is the worst.

You might not think of your skin as an organ; after all, it hardly resembles a kidney or a heart. But the skin is, in fact, the largest organ of the body. It's a natural-growing, one-person army of protection, germ warfare, and elimination. If something happens to the skin, the rest of your body is much more vulnerable to infection, shock, and disease. A burn is the skin's worst nightmare, and unless you act fast, a burn can seep into the skin and invade your entire body.

The Three Goals in Treating All Burns

When it comes to burns, there is a silver lining. The fact is that burns can be treated successfully, if first aid is administered quickly. By reading this section of the book, you'll be ahead of the game. You'll know how to act fast in case of emergency, and you'll know how to treat a burn, regardless of its degree (from first, the least serious, to third, the most damaging) or cause, while you wait for help to arrive.

Remember, the three main objectives to keep in mind when treating burns are:

1. Prevent shock.

2. Ease the pain.

3. Reduce the risk of infection.

The Burn Treatment Commandments

The first aid measures you *don't* take can be as important as those you do take, especially when it comes to burns. For example, earlier in this chapter you learned that treating bruises is different from treating cuts, despite the fact that you can follow basic, general outlines for both. In short, there are always exceptions to every rule. And, when it comes to burns, these exceptions can save a life. Here's the short list on what not to do:

➤ Do not pierce or open blisters. It leaves the burned person "wide open" for infection.

➤ Do not peel off burned dead skin. It not only leaves the new skin underneath too vulnerable to infection, but it can cause scarring.

➤ Do not attempt to peel away any clothing stuck to the burn. Pulling away the cloth can also peel away any healing skin. And, as anyone who's ever had a bandage pulled off knows, it can hurt, too.

➤ Do not use butter, antiseptic creams, or any other "folk remedies" on burns. They can actually cause the infection you're trying to avoid. None of these remedies (especially not butter) will do anything beneficial for major burns.

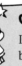

Ouch!

It's one thing to fantasize yourself a hero, but unless you're a trained firefighter or medical professional, you should leave the saving to those who know how. Backdrafts, fallen rafters, smoke inhalation, and related hazards can affect you—instead of being a hero, you may become a victim. The best heroic deed is to get help fast.

In the First Degree

First-degree burns are the most benign and most common burns of all. Accidentally touching a hot burner, getting too much tropical sun, and holding a scalding pot are all ways you can get first-degree burns. However, because first-degree burns irritate nerve endings (especially finger-tips), they can hurt a great deal.

First-degree burns result in red skin (as well as a howling sufferer). There won't be any blisters on a first-degree burn, nor will the skin be broken. There may be some swelling on and around the burned area. Luckily, healing is very quick because only the outermost layer of skin is affected.

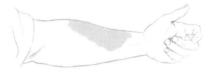

First-degree burns have slight redness or discoloration, along with a bit of swelling and pain.

First-degree burns do not usually need professional medi-cal attention. Simply cool the burn under cold, running water for several minutes to stop the burn from getting worse. You can give the injured person an aspirin (if he or she has no medical complications) and soothe the area with some aloe vera ointment or burn cream.

Second-Degree Burns

By the very nature of their place on the "burn hierarchy," these burns require some medical treatment. You can get a second-degree burn from too much sun; scalding soup, coffee, or tea; or quick flash burns from gasoline or kero-sene lamps.

Second-degree burns are distinguished by the blistery, red, blotchy marks they leave on skin. Blisters form in these burns because the burn penetrates deeper into the layers of skin, releasing body fluids that erupt and cause blisters on the surface. Sometimes the burned area will swell or ooze, and it's painful.

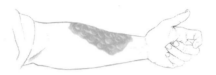

Second-degree burns look red or mottled, and they generally have blisters. These burns may ooze or swell.

Pain from second-degree burns can be vastly reduced by preventing air from getting at those tender, exposed nerve endings and tissues. Here's the best emergency first aid, step-by-step:

1. Submerge the burned area in cold water (as cold as possible). If the burn occurred on the chest or back, pour cold water from a bucket or a hose directly onto the burn.

2. Keep the cold water on the burn until medical help arrives. Try to keep the burn in cold water for at least five minutes.

3. You can also apply a cool, wet cloth to the affected area—but only if you wrap the dressing in plastic first. Cloth tends to adhere to burns, and it can worsen the pain if a physician has to pull it off to treat the burn.

Burns in the Third Degree

Third-degree burns are serious—deadly serious. If you encounter someone who has a third-degree burn, get medical attention fast.

How do you know a third-degree burn from a first- or second-degree one? The injured person looks burnt—the skin is charred and white. Third-degree burns destroy all of the layers of skin (sometimes quite obviously).

First Things First
Did you know that third-degree burns hardly ever hurt at all, at least not initially? That's because nerve endings have been completely burned—the brain can't receive the painful message.

Third-degree burns come from situations like the ones you read about in the paper—where firefighters are rushing from burning buildings and people are rolling on the ground with their clothes on fire. You can also suffer serious burns and shock from pots of boiling water spilling on vulnerable skin or accidents involving electrical outlets.

If the burned person shows any signs of shock, immediately treat that before taking care of the burn. See Chapter 2 for step-by-step instructions on treating shock.

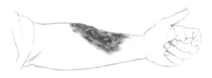

Third-degree burns look like deep wounds and often appear to be white and charred.

As we've already mentioned, third-degree burns are the most severe of all burns. They require medical treatment and precise first aid care. If you know what you're doing, you can help prevent infection from spreading.

1. Call for medical attention if access is immediately available.

2. Treat for shock, if necessary. This is especially true if the burn is caused by electric shock (see the last section of this chapter).

3. If you suspect chemical burning, especially from dangerous acids, you need to take first aid care one step further in order to stop the burn from spreading. As soon as you've called for medical help, pick up the phone and call the local poison control center. As with any type of poison ingestion, inhalation, or burn, these specialists can tell you exactly what you need to do. (See Chapter 12 for more on poisoning.)

4. Remove any tight clothing or jewelry that's nearby but not on the actual burned area. With third-degree burns there's always the danger of swelling, which can cause blood vessels to constrict and create other complications.

5. You can submerge the burned area under cold running water, but avoid ice. Too much cold can exacerbate shock.

6. Pat the area dry and place a very loose sterile cloth over the area to keep away bacteria.

7. If hands are burned, elevate them, keeping them higher than the heart. This can be done by gently placing pillows under the injured person's arms.

8. Burned legs and feet should also be elevated to keep blood flowing smoothly.

9. Keep the injured person still. Do not let him or her walk around.

10. If the face is burned, keep checking for breathing complications. If airways seem to be blocked, follow the instructions in Chapter 2 for performing mouth-to-mouth resuscitation.

11. Above all, get the burn victim to a hospital. Third-degree-burn victims are prime candidates for infection, pneumonia, and other complications, and they need medical attention fast.

A Burn by Any Other Name

Whether the burn is caused by overexposure to the sun, chemical acids, corrosives, or fire, it's the degree of the burn that counts—not the cause. Do keep in mind, however, that chemical burns are more complicated than those that result from fire. Certain acids need to be neutralized in order to prevent the burn from spreading and to prevent a lesser burn from developing into a third-degree burn.

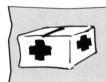

First Things First
When in doubt, treat all burns as if they were third-degree burns.

Dealing with Electric Shock

Electricity causes burns via the flow of electric voltage through the skin. But electric shock can cause more than burns. Bad shocks can cause deep tissue damage, and extremely high voltages may even stop the heart. You can tell an electric shock burn from other burns by the small, discolored marks on the skin at the points of entry and exit of the electricity.

The rest of this chapter deals with handling emergencies involving electric shock, including steps to ensure your safety and help the injured person.

First, Turn Off the Power—If You Can

Before you can administer first aid to a person experiencing an electric shock, you must turn off the power, if you can. Don't waste time on appliance switches or plugs— they might have loose connections, which could have caused the problem in the first place. The best solution? If you're in the house, immediately move to the master fuse and turn off all the power.

Sometimes the situations that cause electric shocks are very simple (such as dropping a hair dryer into the bathtub). But electric shocks don't always occur in the bathroom or kitchen. Sometimes a live wire can fall on a person out-doors, in which case there's no way to shut the power off. Call for help; while you're waiting, you can also do a few things to help—without injuring yourself.

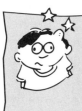

Ouch!
Never try to pull a person away from the electrical current. If you do, you too will become a conductor and the current will run from that person's body into yours.

➤ Stand on a thick pile of newspapers or a fat rubber "welcome mat"—but only as long as it's not raining and the ground is dry. Moisture would immediately make you a conductor regardless of what you're standing on.

➤ Using a wooden broom, mop, or pole, try to push
   the injured person off the live wire or try to push
   the live wire off the injured person.

Always make sure the mat, the pole, and your hands are
dry. The dry, insulated material you're standing on will
prevent the electricity from flowing into you. When
you've turned off the power source that caused the shock,
or you've otherwise moved the power away from the injured person, you can help him or her to safety and get
help.

Treating for Electric Shock Before Help Arrives

Before beginning first aid care, remember to call for emergency help and, as always, practice the universal safety
guidelines discussed in Chapter 1.

1. Because shock is more of a risk with electricity than
   any other type of burn, check the injured person's
   ABCs (see Chapter 1) and take the appropriate measures. If the person is not breathing, immediately begin mouth-to-mouth resuscitation as you learned in
   Chapter 2.

2. While waiting for help, apply a small amount of
   antibacterial or antiburn ointment on the points of
   entry and exit of the electricity.

3. Keep the injured person on his or her back, with the
   feet and legs elevated.

4. If the injured person is unconscious, gently turn
   him or her to the side, supporting the head with a
   pillow. This will aid breathing and keep shock damage from increasing.

5. Gently cover the injured person with a blanket.

Chapter 6

"Help! I'm Choking!"

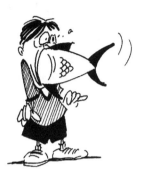

In This Chapter

➤ Recognizing the signs of choking before it's too late

➤ Doing the Heimlich Maneuver

➤ Treating an infant who has swallowed something that's blocking the main airway

It happens so quickly. You're enjoying a nice dinner when, without warning, your companion starts coughing, turns red, and cannot talk. Or maybe you're at home when a baby gets his or her hands on some pennies that just happen to look good enough to eat. Suddenly, someone is choking.

When a person is choking, he or she has a partially blocked or obstructed airway. In simple terms, that means he or she cannot breathe, and first aid must be administered *fast*.

This chapter shows you how to recognize when someone is choking and also explains how to react under various conditions, such as when an infant is choking.

Signs and Symptoms of Choking

Choking can cause as much panic in the observer as in the person actually going through it. It's terrifying to watch someone who is unable to breathe. But you can't let the panic overtake you. First aid must be administered immediately.

Most of us can easily recognize the signs of choking:

➤ Gasping for breath

➤ Grabbing at the throat, mouth agape

➤ Garbled, hoarse speaking

➤ Clammy skin or sweating

➤ Dizziness

➤ Face turning red and tongue becoming swollen

➤ Unconsciousness

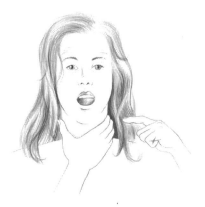

This is the universal sign for choking. Use it if you're choking; provide help if you see someone else using it.

The most effective treatment for choking is the Heimlich Maneuver. If you or someone nearby demonstrates the universal sign for choking or shows any of the warning signals listed above, act quickly. Begin the Heimlich Maneuver, which you'll learn in the next section.

Guide to the Heimlich Maneuver

Although it might sound like a military strategy, the Heimlich Maneuver is the creation of U.S. surgeon Henry J. Heimlich, M.D., whose simple and innovative technique became popular during the 1960s and is now required by law to be prominently displayed on a poster in public places.

The Heimlich Maneuver is a means of dislodging the food or object that is causing breathing problems. It involves hitting the back of an adult to loosen the object, and then applying pressure to the stomach.

If someone appears to be choking, ask him or her directly, "Are you choking?" If the person is crying, coughing, or even wheezing out, "I can't breathe," let him or her try to dislodge the object without intervention. A good, solid cough can do more than your manipulations.

Ouch!
If the person choking becomes unconscious, try mouth-to-mouth resuscitation between Heimlich Maneuver cycles and do everything you can to get medical help—fast.

Use the Heimlich Maneuver immediately only if breathing has stopped or if the person cannot even call for help. If the person can nod—even if he or she can't talk or cough—call for help first, then follow these steps to perform the Heimlich Maneuver:

1. Stand behind the choking victim.

2. Place one hand around the chest for support.

3. Lower the victim's head.

4. Using the heel of your free hand, hit the victim's back hard, between the shoulder blades.

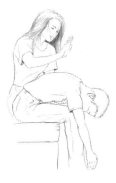

Try dislodging the object with blows to the back.

5. Repeat the above steps rapidly four times.

If steps 1 through 4 do not dislodge the obstructing object and the person continues to choke, follow the remaining steps:

6. Put your arms around the injured person's torso, between the waist and the ribs, as shown on the far left in the following illustration.

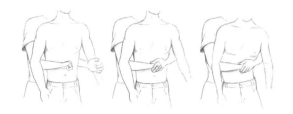

Wrap your arms around the person and apply pressure by thrusting in an inward and upward motion.

7. Place one hand on the torso with your thumb facing the stomach; with your other hand, grab the wrist of your first hand (as in the middle drawing).

8. Pull inward and upward hard four times in rapid succession (as in the right-hand drawing).

9. If the object is still lodged, don't give up. Repeat all eight steps until medical help arrives.

Heimlich Maneuvers for Special Situations

Infants can't tell you they can't breathe. But if they are coughing and crying, it's a good indication that they are not choking. Let them try to work the object out themselves, but be on guard.

If a baby's cough or cry is faint or nonexistent, first aid must be given. The Heimlich Maneuver is slightly different for infants under 18 months of age.

1. First open the baby's mouth. If you can see the object that is causing the choking and you can reach it, perform the "finger sweep" to clean the mouth.

First Aids

The *finger sweep* is a technique you can use
if the object causing the choking is visible.
Put on protective gloves, open the mouth,
and if you can see the object, literally sweep your
fingers in the throat area, using gentle, feather-soft
movements to "rake" up the object and remove it.
Note: *Never* reach blindly into a choking victim's
mouth. You can end up forcing the object down
farther.

2. If you can't see the obstruction, place the baby face
   down on your forearm, with your hand supporting
   the head (as shown in the first drawing in the following illustration).

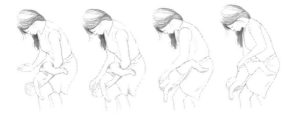

The Heimlich Maneuver for an infant.

3. As you would with an adult, give the same four
   "hits" with the heel of your hand—more gently, of
   course (see the second drawing).

4. Turn the baby to face you. Use both forearms and
   hold the head in the cup of your hand (see the third
   drawing).

5. Using only your fingertips, press down on the baby's
   chest four times (as shown in the fourth drawing).

6. Repeat the procedure until help comes.

Pregnant women and obese persons also need special care. The blows to the back remain the same, using the heel of the hand. However, when you put your arms around them for the inward and upward thrusts, you must adapt to the excess weight. Instead of thrusting between the waist and ribs, push your hands against the breastbone.

Saving Yourself

What if *you* happen to be the person who chokes on a chicken bone, and there's no one around to help? Don't worry. The Heimlich Maneuver is so versatile, you can even perform it on yourself.

1. First dial the phone, knock on the wall, honk the horn—do anything to get help.

2. Lean over the back of a chair.

3. Push your stomach against the top of the chair back as hard as you can.

4. Repeat until help arrives.

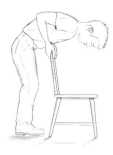

If you must, you can do the Heimlich Maneuver on yourself.

Strange Swallowed Objects

Swallowing small objects is usually not harmful. (Just ask any dog who's been left in the house alone!) Usually, there will be some discomfort as the object passes through the digestive tract, but, eventually, it will be expelled.

In certain circumstances, however, you should call for medical attention immediately: for example, if the swallowed object is sharp and dangerous, such as a needle, a sharp fish bone, a broken chicken bone, or an open safety pin. Likewise, you should seek help if the victim experiences excessive drooling or very severe pain that lasts longer than five minutes.

Chapter 7

Natural Disasters: Drowning and Smoke Inhalation

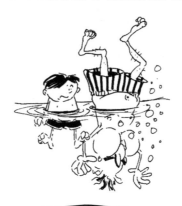

In This Chapter

➤ Rescuing someone who has been over-come by smoke or water—without hurting yourself

➤ Reviving someone who has swallowed too much water

➤ Rescues on ice: The dangers of hypothermia

➤ The signs that indicate when smoke in-halation is a life-or-death situation

One of the most common causes of accidental death in the United States is drowning. Drowning doesn't just happen in oceans, lakes, or half-frozen ponds. You can drown in a bathtub—or even in a wading pool.

Sometimes drowning occurs as a result of another injury—a heart attack or stroke that causes unconsciousness. Sometimes people drown by diving into water that's too shallow and suffering a head injury. And sometimes muscle cramps cause panic, which in turn leads to drowning.

Smoke, like water, is something we come in contact with every day. Air pollution, smog, secondhand (or firsthand) cigarette smoke—we draw smoke into our lungs with every breath.

This chapter offers steps you can take to help rescue a drowning person or someone overcome by smoke. We provide the first aid steps you should follow to resuscitate a rescued drowning victim. We also teach you how to rescue someone in a burning house or in a smoke-filled room, when you don't even have any air to breathe.

Water Rescue

The signs for help are easy to identify. A cry, splashing, and a period of immersion when the person disappears from sight—these are all signs that someone in the water may be a drowning victim.

The larger the body of water, the more difficult the rescue. Still, when the rescuer knows what he or she is doing, a rescue is possible.

1. If a lifeguard is nearby, let him or her do the rescuing. Otherwise, shout for help as loud as you can.

2. Try to reach the injured person without leaving the shore. Use your arm, your leg, a sweatshirt, a life

preserver, a rope, a rescue pole, or anything that floats.

Ouch!

Oceans are vast places with strong currents and tides. If you're on the beach and spot someone drowning far out in the water, get help as fast as you can. Though it's frustrating to stand on the sidelines, the odds are against you. If you're not a lifeguard equipped to handle crashing waves, you're likely to become a victim instead of a hero.

3. Hold onto something on solid ground (such as another person) so you aren't swept away by strong currents.

4. If you can't reach the victim from the shore, locate a boat and find someone to assist you. Be sure that you, or someone with you, can operate the craft.

5. When a boat is not available, swim out to the spot where the victim was last seen—but only if you're a good swimmer. Currents, undertow, and cold water can hinder average swimmers. Even if you're a good swimmer, always have a flotation device with you— something that the drowning victim can hold onto as you swim back to shore. If the drowning person is unconscious, hold him or her on the flotation device and use a sidestroke and strong kicks to return to shore.

Ouch!
Never let a drowning person grab onto you in deep water. There's a chance that he or she will drag you under as well. Especially if you're out of shape, don't even attempt to go out into the water. Your best bet is to call for help and accept your fate as a landlubber hero.

When we talk about "personal flotation devices," we're not spewing out some kind of euphemistic, politically correct jargon. Personal flotation devices are life preservers, life jackets, thick floating dinghies, or rafts that can save a life. All of these lightweight devices can keep a person afloat and prevent him or her from drowning. Like car safety belts, personal flotation devices are meant to be preventative. You should use one any time you're out fishing, boating, or swimming (especially for children and weak swimmers).

Reviving the Victim

Suppose you manage to pull a drowning person back to dry land. What do you do next?

Rescuing is only half the job. Reviving someone who was drowning or has swallowed water is the other half and is equally important when it comes to saving a life.

Reviving a person involves performing mouth-to-mouth resuscitation (see Chapter 2). Of course, you should implement universal safety guidelines whenever possible. If you have an airway bag in your first aid kit, use it.

As always, call for help before beginning these important first aid emergency measures.

First Things First

Babies are particularly vulnerable to drowning incidents; because they sometimes don't have enough strength to lift their heads, babies can drown even in wading pools. If you must perform mouth-to-mouth resuscitation on a baby, don't use forceful breaths. Instead, breathe gentle puffs of air four times into the baby's mouth and nose.

1. Turn the drowning person's head to the side, allowing any water to drain from his or her mouth and nose.

2. Turn the head back to the center.

3. Begin mouth-to-mouth resuscitation on land, if possible, or in the water if the injured person needs immediate life-and-death measures. (See Chapter 2 for general resuscitation procedures.)

4. Breathe hard four times into the mouth of the injured person as you pinch his or her nose (see Chapter 2). This helps air get past any water that is clogging the breathing passageways and the lungs.

5. After four strong breaths, put your ear near the mouth, listen for breath, and watch the chest for any breathing movement.

6. Check for a pulse.

7. Repeat the cycle.

You're not out of the water just because the drowning victim starts to breathe and choke. In fact, the first 48 hours after a drowning incident can be the most dangerous. Complications resulting from water exposure—pneumonia, infection, heart failure—can all occur during this time. Therefore, you should always take a drowning victim to the hospital.

Ice Rescue

Ice fishing, skating, and snowmobiling are all dangerous sports because of the possibility of thin, weak ice. Without any warning, ice can crack, and you or your companion can fall through into the icy water. Two major concerns result: First, extremely cold water can cause severe hypothermia and frostbite. Second, a victim can get trapped underneath the ice and drown.

An ice rescue can be a challenge, but it's not impossible if you follow the rules presented next. As always, before beginning these ice rescue rules, call for professional help— either a nearby hospital, ambulance, or even a ranger. It's nice to know that backup aid is on its way while you're teetering around on "thin ice."

Rule #1: Don't step on the breaking ice.

If you do, there will be two of you in need of help.

Rule #2: Reach for the person with a scarf or other clothing item, a tree limb, or a pole.

Using another object to reach the drowning person ensures that you keep your distance from the weak, dangerous ice. If there are others who can aid in the rescue attempt, you can form a human chain to reach the victim. To do so, each person lies face-down on firm ice and holds the ankles of the person in front of him. The "anchor person" should remain on shore, firmly gripping the legs of the first person lying down (and with a rope tied to his torso and a sturdy tree, if possible). The following drawing illustrates this procedure.

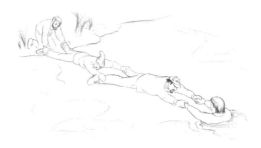

Use a human chain to rescue someone who has fallen through the ice.

Another reliable rescue device is a small inflatable dinghy. Once blown up, it's smooth and sleek enough to get you across the ice to the victim, but light enough not to weigh you down. The dinghy can also be used as a life preserver, helping the victim reach up and out of the freezing water. But before you set out, make sure the ice is strong enough to support your weight. Although the dinghy will keep you afloat if ice breaks, it will be much harder to initiate a rescue.

Rule #3: Slide the drowning person across the ice.

Never carry a victim across a body of water covered in ice—the extra weight can be dangerous if it's concentrated in one spot. If, instead, you slide the person, thereby dispersing the extra weight onto a larger area of the ice, the ice is less likely to crack.

Rule #4: Begin mouth-to-mouth resuscitation.

Don't give up if the individual appears to be dead. Icy water lowers body temperature, which, in turn, slows down all body functions. People have been known to be revived 20 minutes after a drowning incident with no brain or heart damage.

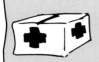

First Things First

Do not give up on a person if, after an hour's search on the ice, you still haven't found him or her. The frigid water slows down the body functions; what would drown a person in the tropics in 5 minutes can take more than 60 minutes in freezing water!

Rule #5: Treat for shock if necessary.

Because of the frigid water, an injured person might be in shock. Cover him or her with a warm blanket to raise body temperature. Although it seems logical to give the person something hot to drink, you should *never* give food or drink to someone semiconscious or suffering from shock. (See Chapter 2 for step-by-step instructions for treating shock.)

Rule #6: Treat for frostbite if necessary.

Frostbite is indicated by red skin, which then changes to a gray color, and ultimately changes to a bright, icy whiteness (a sign of tissue damage). Treat frostbite by gently warming the body parts with lukewarm water. Do not massage the area because this can cause more tissue damage. Chapter 10 gives more details on treating hypothermia and frostbite.

Shock vs. Hypothermia

Shock and hypothermia might sound like completely different conditions, but they both present many of the same symptoms and can both lead to the same dire results. (See Chapter 2 for detailed first aid care for shock.)

Mild hypothermia occurs when body temperature drops below 98 degrees but remains above 90 degrees. Symptoms include:

➤ Mumbled speech

➤ Chills

➤ Clumsy finger movement

➤ Lack of coordination

➤ Skin numbness

➤ Weakness

➤ Shivering

➤ Mild confusion

Severe hypothermia occurs when body temperature drops below 90 degrees. Shivering might stop completely, but in its stead are:

➤ Paralysis

➤ Irregular heartbeat

➤ Inability to walk or stand

➤ Unconsciousness, which can lead to death

Ouch!

Popular first aid treatment for hypothermia used to call for one vital element: an ambulance to get the victim to the hospital quickly. Not any longer. Today, health professionals know that any movement can cause irregular heartbeats, endangering the heart of the person suffering from hypothermia. Even emergency medical teams know to warm up the victim first. When they succeed in getting body temperature above 90 degrees, they move him or her to a hospital.

If you think these symptoms sound like those of shock, you're right. Both can cause mental and physical dysfunction. Both can lead to death. A major difference, however, is that shock results from trauma that can occur in any climate; hypothermia is directly related to body temperature and cold.

Treatment for hypothermia includes giving the person hot liquids to drink, covering up the entire body with warm blankets, and generally getting the victim as warm as possible. The key is to get the body temperature back up and to get the victim out of the "cold zone." Just don't buy into the St.-Bernard-as-rescue-dog myth—liquor can mess up body temperature regulation. Your brain will trick you into feeling like your body temperature is rising, when it's not.

Smoke Signals

Obviously, smoke is a by-product of fire, but you don't have to be locked up in an unventilated burning room to be overcome by smoke. Smoke inhalation also can occur from minor fires, such as:

➤ Fireplaces with faulty air ducts

➤ Stovetop fires

➤ The smoldering at the onset of electrical fires

➤ Broiler fires

➤ Grill fires in improperly ventilated porches and decks

➤ Smoldering furniture or mattresses (which can occur if a smoker fails to put out his or her matches or cigarettes)

Minor Smoke Inhalation

The signs of smoke inhalation vary. Minor problems include irritated eyes, coughing jags, and general weakness—which can turn into more serious symptoms if the victim doesn't get away from the smoke.

To treat smoke inhalation, follow these steps:

1. First, get the victim into the fresh air.

2. Have the victim sit down until he or she begins to feel better.

3. After coughing has subsided, offer a glass of water to calm a burning throat.

4. Place a cool washcloth over the victim's eyes and forehead.

Minor incidents don't usually require special medical care. Trust your instincts and your methods of observation. If the person seems fine and doesn't have a lingering cough, he or she will not need immediate medical attention. But it's always a good idea to call the family physician and have him or her give the "all clear."

Ouch!

Although minor incidents are not medical emergencies, they can turn into emergencies if the person involved has asthma, allergic bronchitis, emphysema, or any other chronic pulmonary disease. These people are more sensitive to smoke, and what is minor to a hardier person can wreak havoc for a sensitive one. Even smoke from an ordinary campfire can cause a severe asthma attack. A good rule of thumb is to seek medical attention for any asthmatic who is wheezing, no matter how minor the inhalation seems. This especially holds true for young children.

Serious Smoke Inhalation

Symptoms of serious smoke inhalation requiring first aid include:

➤ Continued wheezing and coughing

➤ An inability to breathe

➤ Choking

➤ Lightheadedness

➤ Ash, black char, or smoke around the mouth and nose

➤ Weakness and lethargy that could lead to unconsciousness

To treat a serious case of smoke inhalation, in which the victim is suffering from the symptoms described above, follow these steps:

1. Call for help.

2. Drag the injured person away from the smoke.

3. Check the victim's breathing. If he or she is having difficulty, perform mouth-to-mouth resuscitation (or CPR, if trained) until help arrives. (See Chapter 2 for more information.)

First Things First

Calling for aid first is an insurance benefit. Just in case you also are overcome by the smoke, someone will be on the way to help.

4. Cover the victim with a blanket. If he or she is lying on the cold ground, place a blanket underneath as well.

5. Loosen clothes around the neck and torso to help breathing.

6. To prevent possible shock, make sure the victim is lying on his or her back, with a pillow behind the head if he or she is having difficulty breathing, or a pillow elevating the legs and feet if all seems well.

7. If the victim is unconscious, turn his or her head to the side to prevent possible vomit from choking him or her.

Don't Get Burned: A Safe Rescue

In case you have to dart into the fire to rescue someone, here are some tips to ensure your safe return. First of all, remember that you shouldn't go in a burning room or building solo if you can help it. Have someone wait for you outside. Otherwise, you could become hurt, instead of a hero. And always call for professional help first. If possible, wait until the fire truck arrives. Firefighters know how to get in and out of a burning building much better than you do. They also have the equipment to handle electrical fires, wood-burning fires, and chemical fires— and they know how to use it.

First Things First

If you're caught in a fire, the first thing you should do is cover your face with a wet towel, a piece of cloth, your shirt, or anything else you can find to help reduce the inhalation of smoke. You cannot save a life or yourself if you're overcome with smoke, too.

If you can't possibly wait for help, there are some safety measures you can take. If the smoke in a room is not too thick, take several deep breaths before entering. Then, holding your breath, enter and pull the victim outside. If smoke is heavy, determine whether it's circling the ceiling (which is usually the case because heat and warm air rise) or hanging around the floor (which can occur in chemical fires). Then enter the room accordingly. Crouch if the smoke is high. Stand tall and keep your head up if it's low.

By the time you and the victim are out in the fresh air, the fire department should have arrived—hopefully. Don't compromise yourself further by trying to put the fire out on your own. Let the professionals do their jobs.

First Things First

If you're still waiting for help at the scene of a fire, forget the building and concentrate on the survivors. Remember the "stop, drop, and roll" method to help someone whose clothing is ablaze:

1. Stop in your tracks.

2. Drop to the ground.

3. Roll around on the ground to smother the flames.

Chapter 8

Ear, Eye, and Nose Damage Control

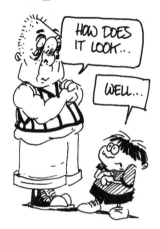

Knowing how to administer first aid to the ears, the eyes, and the nose is one of the most important tools you can learn—by doing so, you can literally give back to a person the sense of being alive. This chapter presents the basic first aid techniques for dealing with ear, eye, and nose injuries.

Ear Aid

If a person's ear is bleeding after he or she has suffered a blow to the head and the person is unconscious, immediate medical attention is necessary (see Chapter 9, "Head Injuries, Heart Attacks, and Strokes"). If the person is conscious, you should inspect the ear to look for the source of the bleeding and treat the injury accordingly.

Ouch!
Don't reach for ear drops every time someone complains of an earache—you could possibly cause more damage. If the earache is the result of a foreign object in the ear, the medicine could intensify pain and spread damage.

Sometimes an ear injury can look worse than it really is; a surface cut can cause profuse bleeding and can appear to be serious, but you should treat the injury only for what it is— a cut. (To stop bleeding, follow the steps in Chapter 2.) Once you've ruled out simple cuts or head injuries, you can begin ear aid.

Before we get into some of the injuries that can occur in the ear, let's go over the three NEVERs in ear first aid care. When you're helping someone with an ear injury, make sure you:

➤ Never put anything inside a damaged ear.

➤ Never try to stop the bleeding. This is one case when bleeding is encouraged. If you try to stop it, the blood can back up and seep into the inner ear. Stuffing cotton balls in the ear to clot fluids is a definite no-no!

➤ Never shake, jiggle, or thump a person's head to restore hearing. Contrary to what you might see in cartoons, people are not pinball machines.

Against the Tide: Swimmer's Ear

Contrary to popular belief, swimmer's ear—that uncomfortable, swollen feeling with the accompanying "swishing" sound—does not come from too much water in the ear or from eardrum damage caused by too much swimming. It's an inflammation or infection of the outer ear canal. Swimmer's ear can be caused by bacteria, or, like athlete's foot, it can also be a fungus.

The main symptom of swimmer's ear is pain, with possible swelling, redness, and itchiness. Over time, the ear can become clogged, resulting in a loss of hearing. There can also be a drainage of pus from the ear.

You should make an appointment with your doctor; in the meantime, there are a few things you can do to ease the pain of swimmer's ear:

➤ Place a heating pad (set to medium) on the ear to help ease the soreness.

➤ Sit up as much as possible, even propping yourself up in bed with pillows. This allows blood to drain away from the ears so there's less "stuffiness."

➤ Drink lots of water and juice. Liquids not only help "flush" away infection, but the act of swallowing helps clear your ear canals.

➤ Chew gum. Chewing a piece of gum or food (and yawning) also helps clear the ear canals and ease the pain.

➤ Take an over-the-counter anti-inflammatory medication such as Motrin or Advil. Tylenol, too, will help control the pain.

A Pierced Eardrum

A pierced eardrum happens more often than you might think. It can result from a cotton swab pushed too far into the ear, a super loud noise, or a shift in pressure on the eardrum (like when you dive into very deep water).

The main symptoms of a pierced eardrum are loss of hearing and pain. If you or someone you're with experiences these symptoms, you should call for medical help immediately. You might also see some blood draining from the ear; if so, treat it in this way:

1. Cover the ear with a sterile gauze pad.

2. Tape the pad down loosely but securely.

3. Position the injured person on his or her side with the damaged ear toward the ground to encourage drainage. (Blood that pools in the ear can cause more hearing loss and possible infection.)

Ouch!

If wax accumulation has reached a point at which it actually hinders your hearing, you'll need more than just a cotton swab to clean your ears—if you attempt to swab your ears, you may even end up doing more damage.

Foreign Objects in Foreign Places

Although it sounds crazy, an insect buzzing around your head can fly into your ear and become stuck. And insects are only one of the many foreign objects that can enter the ear and cause damage. Many children also have the delightful habit of testing out their nimble fingers and dexterity on tiny toys, jacks, beads, food, or coins and putting them compactly and complacently in their ears.

Here's a step-by-step guide to removing foreign objects from the ear:

1. If the object is a live insect, put a drop or two of mineral oil, baby oil, or vegetable oil in the ear canal. The oil will kill the insect.

2. If you can clearly see the object in the person's ear, remove it carefully with a pair of tweezers, but only if the object is near the surface.

3. If you cannot see the object clearly or if it's lodged in the ear canal, tilt the sufferer's head to the same side as the injured ear.

4. Gently shake his or her head in this position.

5. If this doesn't work, leave the victim alone. Attempting to remove a deep or embedded object can damage the ear. Call for professional help.

Even if you get the foreign object out of the ear, you should seek medical help. With an *otoscope* (an instrument that magnifies the eardrum), a professional can determine whether all the material has been removed.

Eye Injuries

As I'm sure you well know, even an eyelash in your eye can be very painful. So an eye injury such as a larger foreign object in the eye, a black eye, or a cut on the cornea is definitely cause for medical attention.

The main point is that you should get help quickly. Go to your private physician, a medicenter, or an emergency room—just don't waste any time getting there.

There's a Fly in My Eye!

Flecks of dirt, bugs, and eyelashes all irritate the eyes. Of course, they usually feel much bigger than they are: A grain of sand can feel like a stone. In addition to pain and irritation, a foreign object in the eye can also cause redness, a stinging sensation when the person blinks, and sudden light sensitivity.

Your first instinct may be to rub your eye to try to get rid of the pain. But this can have the opposite effect. Rubbing your eye can dig the dirt in deeper, causing more damage and making the debris even harder to remove.

Ouch!

If a foreign object in the eye affects the victim's vision, emergency medical aid is especially important. Particularly if a person experiences blurred vision or sees waves, specks of light, or blackness, he or she needs immediate attention.

Follow these instructions to remove an object that you can see in another person's eye:

1. Flush the eye with cool, clean water. If you're not near a sink, use a pitcher, a glass, or an eyedropper. If the object is lying on the surface of the eyeball, the flushing action should remove the object.

2. If you can still see the object on the eye and it does not flush out with the water, gently cover BOTH eyes with gauze pads (there's less eye movement when it's dark), and seek help as fast as you can.

If you cannot see anything in the injured person's eye, an object might be stuck under the eyelid. Follow these steps to treat that type of eye injury:

1. Flush the eye with cool, clean water. If flushing the eye doesn't alleviate the pain, you'll have to use your hands—wash them first to prevent infection.

2. Place the injured person under a good light (or anchor a flashlight so that you can see into the eye and still use both hands).

3. Have the person look up, and gently pull down the lower lid. If you can see a particle on the inside of the lower lid or at the lower edge of the eyeball, flush it out with an eyedropper or gently touch a wet Q-tip or a moistened gauze strip or handkerchief to the particle so that it adheres to the cotton.

4. If the particle doesn't stick to the Q-tip with a gentle touch, don't keep trying—you can cause more damage. Cover the eyes with gauze pads and get medical help.

5. If the particle sticks to the Q-tip, remove it and rinse the eye with cool water.

6. If you can't see anything on the lower lid, check the upper one. Curl the lashes and upper lid over a Q-tip, and be careful not to pull.

7. If you see an object on the upper lid or on the upper surface of the eyeball, follow the above directions to remove the particle.

Ouch!

Chlorine and salt water can irritate eyes and contact lenses. If you're going swimming, it's best to take your lenses out *before* you go into the water. You can purchase swimming goggles that have prescription lenses, if necessary.

Eye Scream: Cuts and Scratches

Think of *any* cut or scratch on the eye as serious, and treat it as a medical emergency. Call for help; while you're driving the injured person to a doctor, keep him or her in a semireclining position. Place a pillow beneath the head, if necessary. Cover both eyes with sterile gauze pads held in place with long strips of adhesive tape.

Now for the list of DON'Ts. The following list explains what you should avoid when treating cuts or scratches on the eyeball, the eyelids, or even the skin around the eyes:

➤ Don't exert pressure on the eye to stop bleeding. Although it may look bad, eye bleeding is rarely dangerous, and pressure will only cause more damage to the delicate eye area.

➤ Don't attempt to remove contact lenses even if they are causing the injured person excessive pain. This too will exert pressure on the eye, which in turn can cause more damage.

➤ Don't let the injured person rub his or her eye. It will cause more irritation.

➤ Don't flush the eye with water. Bleeding, especially with loss of vision, can mean damage to the eyeball, a condition that water can further irritate.

When Chemicals Get in Your Eyes

When some chemicals get in the eye, they can cause burns, terrible pain, and even blindness. Some of the chemicals that can burn the eye include:

➤ Acid

➤ Enzyme products used for clogged drains

➤ Bleach

➤ Bathroom and kitchen cleaners

➤ Ammonia

➤ Furniture oils

➤ Hair dye

➤ Alcohol

When a person gets a chemical in his or her eye, it's an emergency that requires immediate first aid. Follow these steps to administer the appropriate first aid treatment:

1. Tilt the injured person's head to the same side as the injured eye. (You don't want the chemicals to get in the good eye as well.)

2. Gently open the damaged eye the best that you can with the fingers of one hand.

3. With the other hand, pour cool water into the eye. (You can also use cool milk.)

4. Keep pouring water in the eye until help arrives. The more you flush the eye, the better the chance that the chemical will wash out and no permanent damage will be done.

First Things First
Always keep an extra contact lens case, filled with fresh solution, in your purse, attaché case, or pocket. This way, if a dot of mascara or a fleck of dirt gets into your eye and onto your contact lens, forcing you to remove the lens, you'll have a sterile place to store it.

A Black Eye

A black eye usually looks worse than it really is (emotional pain aside). Whether it's the result of a punch, walking into a wall, or even extreme suction caused by tight goggles while swimming, a black eye needs medical attention. Sometimes there is bleeding that's not outwardly apparent. Likewise, the injury that caused the black eye may have also caused a contact lens to scratch the cornea. And if the black eye is accompanied by swelling, the swelling may affect a person's vision.

Sometimes a blow to the eye will cause swelling without those "attractively colored hues." Treat swelling as you would discoloration. A bruise is a bruise is a bruise, whatever color it may be.

The best first aid is to take the injured person to a medical professional and let him or her take a look at the eye. While you're waiting:

1. Make sure the injured person is lying comfortably on his or her back.

2. Have the injured person keep his or her eyes shut. If necessary, cover both eyes with a sterile gauze pad.

3. Soak a washcloth, a gauze pad, or any available piece of cloth in cold water, and place the wet compress over the closed eyes to ease discomfort.

The Nose Knows: Nosey Nosebleeds

Sure, if you get punched in the nose, it's very likely that you'll end up with a bloody nose. But what about spontaneous nosebleeds—those sudden, worrisome bouts that seem to come from nowhere? Don't worry. In most cases, those seemingly unprovoked nosebleeds are more annoying than dangerous.

Technically, a nosebleed occurs when the tissue lining the inside of the nose becomes irritated. These irritations can be caused by any of the following things:

➤ A dry nose caused by colds and sinus medicine

➤ Excessive blowing from colds, flus, and allergies

➤ Too much picking

➤ Excessive use of nasal sprays

If someone around you suddenly gets a nosebleed, don't panic. Follow these steps for treatment:

1. If possible, have the injured person sit in a chair, leaning forward very slightly. (Leaning forward keeps blood from going down the throat and causing respiratory problems.)

2. Make sure the person doesn't swallow any blood; it can make him or her gag or vomit. Instead, ask the victim to spit out any blood that pools in the mouth.

3. Place a cold cloth on the nose. Have the person apply pressure on the nostrils with the thumb and forefinger, pinching the nostrils tightly for at least 10 minutes. If the victim is too weak to do so, apply the pressure yourself (taking care to wear protective gloves).

4. When the cloth begins to become warm, rewet it with more cold water.

5. After 10 minutes, slowly let go of the nose. If bleeding continues, roll two small pads of gauze to fit into each nostril. Insert them into the nose, making sure the ends of the gauze strips stick out for easy removal.

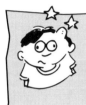

Ouch!

Do not use cotton balls or Band-Aids as pads for bleeding nostrils. They will stick to the inside of the nose and cause more irritation and bleeding.

6. Pinch the nostrils for another 10 minutes.

7. Remove the gauze pads. If the person's nose is still bleeding, seek medical assistance.

Chapter 9

Head Injuries, Heart Attacks, and Strokes

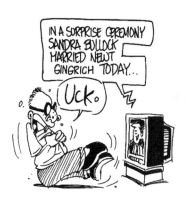

IN A SURPRISE CEREMONY SANDRA BULLOCK MARRIED NEWT GINGRICH TODAY...

Uck.

In This Chapter

➤ Recognizing the signs of a concussion

➤ Recognizing the symptoms of a possible heart attack

➤ The difference between a stroke and a heart attack—and how to treat them

More than 500,000 people suffer from head injuries every day, most of which are the result of car, bike, and motorcycle accidents and falls. Because today's technology is so advanced, people who would have once been pronounced DOA due to head injuries are now able to continue living functional, full lives. But that's only possible if a person receives help right away and begins rehabilitation quickly.

Coronary heart disease is the leading cause of death in this country, and strokes come in as the third leading cause of death. We're not asking you to dwell on these conditions. But, like animal bites or bumps on the head, they can happen to you or someone around you when you least expect it—and you should know what to do in such situations. Armed with the information in this chapter, you could help save a life.

Head Injury: Bump or Concussion?

Depending on the power of the "bang" and the location, a brain injury can be anything from a minor bump that goes away in a few days to a severe head injury that leaves the victim lying in a coma for a long time. Most head injuries are closed—this means that an observer can't see any blood, bumps, or bruises, but it doesn't mean that all those things aren't occurring inside the skull. You must, therefore, rely on your powers of observation. Look for signs that are similar to any illness: nausea, chills, shock, dizziness, and disorientation.

A Bump Is a Lump

If a person merely bumps his or her head on, say, a cabinet door or a dresser drawer, chances are it will hurt, but the pain will soon subside. The person might have a headache and even a lump where the bump happened, but there shouldn't be any other symptoms. An ice compress and some aspirin should do the trick, especially when combined with a small nap (which will stop movement for a while).

If the bump doesn't subside within 24 hours and/or if the person experiences nausea, chills, dizziness, or a spacey feeling that doesn't go away, he or she should call the doctor immediately. It's possible that the victim suffered a more serious concussion.

Concussions

A concussion can be anything from a temporary loss of consciousness to that bell-like "ding" a baseball player will hear for 10 minutes after being socked in the head by a hardball. The effects of a concussion can be a one-time-only reaction, or they can be long-lasting, consisting of several reactions occurring over time. The latter is what happens to "punch-drunk" fighters who become increasingly uncoordinated and eventually become unable to perform in the ring.

If a concussion is suspected, you should always seek medical help. Your physician can determine whether any neurological damage has occurred, and the victim can begin rehabilitation treatment to prevent the damage from increasing. Keep the victim as prone, still, and immobile as possible until you see the doctor.

Skull Fractures

Of course, there are those terrible accidents that do puncture the skull. A bullet or a shard of glass can easily result in a skull fracture and a brain injury. This open head injury puts a person at further risk because of the dangers of infection through the "open door." Treat a skull fracture as a medical emergency, not only because of the seriousness of the blow to the head, but also because of the risk of hemorrhaging and infection.

A Mild Head Injury: Five Good Signs

All head injuries should be taken very seriously, but keep in mind that about 75 percent of all such injuries turn out to have only mild consequences, which is good news. Still, we suggest that you seek medical help for any and all suspected head injuries, just to be certain that all is well and to prevent future problems. When a person has a mild head injury, you'll usually observe the following five conditions:

1. The injured person does not lose consciousness or is out only briefly. He or she may be confused for up to 20 minutes.

2. The person shows only mild physical symptoms of neurological damage, including nausea, dizziness, or blurry vision (which can crop up any time within three months of the accident).

Ouch!
Always seek medical help if a person loses consciousness, even if it's just for a minute or two. Loss of consciousness means that some part of the brain has suffered damage. Early intervention is the best treatment.

3. The person is treated in the emergency room and is not admitted at all, or is hospitalized for no more than a week. He or she is ordered to rest and restrict activity just long enough for the bruised and jolted brain to heal, and for the results of diagnostic tests to show little damage.

4. After three months, the injured person has few side effects.

5. There is no motor damage, and the injured person's faculties (the ability to think and solve problems) are intact.

Treating a Mild Head Injury

Sometimes a head injury can start out minor and become serious a few hours later. If a person gets up and dusts him- or herself off, but then goes home and goes right to sleep, it could be a sign of a more serious condition. If you see that a person is sleeping excessively within 24 hours of a head injury, take him or her to the emergency room.

It's always best to get medical help for any sort of head injury. If a person blacks out, medical attention is imperative—even though it can still signal only a minor head injury. Call for an emergency team quickly. While you are waiting for help to arrive, follow these steps:

1. Immobilize the victim as best you can, keeping the person on his or her back in case of possible spinal problems. (See Chapter 2, "When Emergencies Can't Wait: The Top 10 'How To's.")

2. Avoid giving the victim alcohol, sedatives, or even water.

3. Observe the person for signs of shock and treat accordingly (see Chapter 2).

4. Keep the victim warm.

5. Use ice on the head to ease the pain.

6. If the victim is unconscious, time the length of the blackout. This will help in determining a diagnosis later.

7. If the injured person is released to your care, watch him or her carefully for at least 48 hours. Make sure no symptoms recur. If they do, bring him or her back to the hospital as soon as possible.

Danger Signs of a Serious Head Injury

Unfortunately, the other 25 percent of head injuries cause moderate to serious damage. If the injured person exhibits any of the following symptoms immediately after an accident, he or she probably has a moderate or serious injury:

➤ Unconsciousness for 10 minutes or more

➤ Seizures or convulsions

➤ Inability to swallow or control elimination

 First Aids

A person who is unconscious for more than 24 hours but has steady vital signs is said to be in a *coma*. Although the person appears to be sleeping, studies show that he or she is affected by verbal communication, touching, music, and even a recognized fragrance.

➤ Paralysis

➤ Slurred speech

➤ Loss of memory or confusion that lasts for more than 15 minutes

➤ Personality change, usually in aggressive, violent ways

➤ Difficulty breathing

➤ Pupils of unequal size

If someone around you suffers what appears to be a moderate or serious head injury, first make sure that help is on the way (preferably from a trauma center), and then begin first aid. The next section covers the steps you should take to provide first aid for a serious or life-threatening head injury.

Emergency First Aid for Serious Head Injuries

If you suspect serious head injury, you need to take care of three things right from the start:

1. *Observe* for signs of shock, a concussion, or a skull fracture.

2. *Immobilize* the victim to prevent further damage to either the brain or the spinal cord.

3. *Treat* any bleeding scalp cuts and wounds to avoid infection.

If you're in a situation in which you need to provide first aid care to a person who has experienced a severe head injury, follow these steps:

1. Call for help immediately.

2. See if the injured person is unconscious. Note the length of time the unconsciousness lasts.

3. Look for bleeding from the eyes, nose, or ears (it doesn't have to be bright red blood; it can be a brown discoloration around the rims of the eyes), which can signal internal hemorrhaging. Keep the injured person on his or her back.

4. If the injured person is conscious and does not appear to have a neck injury, place a pillow under the person's head and turn his or her face to the side.

5. While you're waiting for help, treat any scalp wounds. Clean cuts thoroughly, cover them with gauze, and secure the gauze firmly but not too tightly.

Ouch!
Do not give any food or water to a person who has suffered a serious head injury—this could induce vomiting and impede breathing in a semiconscious or unconscious person. Ice packs won't help either. The best medicine is to get the person to a hospital—fast.

6. Look for physical signs of brain injury. These can include:

   - ➤ Severe headaches
   - ➤ Slurred words
   - ➤ Loss of vision or double vision
   - ➤ Bruising behind the ear or around the eyes
   - ➤ Pupils of unequal size
   - ➤ Convulsions
   - ➤ Vomiting
   - ➤ Loss of short-term memory
   - ➤ Clear or bloody fluid seeping from the ear, nose, or mouth
   - ➤ Weakness or paralysis in limbs

7. If any of the signs described in Step 6 appear before an emergency medical team shows up, immobilize the injured person (see Chapter 2). This is crucial for preventing any more damage to the brain, spinal cord, or neck.

8. For at least 48 hours after the injured person has been released from medical care, he or she should be watched for the symptoms described in Step 6. If the symptoms recur, the victim should again seek emergency medical care as quickly as possible.

Warning Signs of a Heart Attack

Heart attacks can be divided into two separate conditions: angina and myocardial infarction.

The temporary pain associated with *angina* can be caused by a spasm in the heart's coronary arteries, which usually occurs when there's inadequate blood flow to the heart. Rest and/or nitroglycerin pills placed under the tongue can halt pain from angina within five minutes. Most people who are prone to angina carry nitroglycerin pills with them at all times. Angina usually occurs during exertion or exercise; if it occurs when a person is at rest, it could be a sign of a possible heart attack. The person should seek medical help immediately.

Myocardial infarction (MI) or *cardiovascular disease (CVS)* are other names for a heart attack. Here, a piece of the heart muscle is actually destroyed when a coronary artery completely "shuts down." Heart attacks do not occur only during periods of overexertion (while shoveling snow, for example); serious heart attacks might occur while a person is at rest, several hours *after* a strenuous experience, exercise, or heavy meal. The symptoms listed below can indicate a heart attack; if a person near you has *any* of these symptoms, call for help and begin first aid measures immediately.

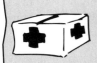

First Things First

It's difficult to describe exactly what pressure or pain in the chest feels like. Some people describe it as a "tightness" or a "crushing feeling," or like a "herd of elephants trampling over my heart."

➤ Uncomfortable pressure, fullness, squeezing, or pain in the center of the chest lasting for more than two minutes

➤ Pain that spreads out to the shoulders, neck, jaw, arms, and stomach

➤ Gasping or shortness of breath that gets worse when lying flat

➤ "Heartburn"-like pain that doesn't improve with antacids

➤ Chest pain combined with lightheadedness, severe anxiety, heavy sweating, pale skin and bluish lips, irregular or rapid pulse, or nausea

Chest pain doesn't always mean a heart attack. In fact, most chest pains aren't heart attacks at all, merely symptoms of indigestion, muscle strain, shingles, or respiratory ailments. If any of the "red flags" appear, however, it's better to be embarrassed in the emergency room than to be, well...dead.

How to Help

Although a heart attack is a frightening proposition, there is good news. With today's sophisticated equipment, procedures, and diagnostic tools for treating heart attacks, people who suffer an attack can go on to live long, productive lives. But the word to remember here is "help." Getting help fast is the only way to possibly prevent disaster. Even if you're sure that the stab of pain you feel is indigestion, go to the doctor. Better to be safe than sorry.

Follow these steps if you think someone is having a heart attack:

1. Call 911 for help immediately.

2. If you know CPR (cardiopulmonary resuscitation), and the victim needs it, begin it immediately. See the information on CPR at the end of this chapter and in Chapter 2 for details.

3. If you don't know CPR, sit the person up or have him or her rest in a semireclining position, whichever is more comfortable.

4. Loosen any restrictive clothing around the neck, such as a collar, tie, shirt, or scarf.

5. Observe and watch the ABCs you learned about in Chapter 1. If the ill person loses consciousness,

continue to check his or her pulse. If he or she vomits, turn the head to the side and clean the mouth.

6. If the ill person has angina medication, place it under his or her tongue (but don't give nitroglycerin pills unless a doctor has prescribed them for that person). If the pain goes away, chances are the person has had an angina attack and will soon be fine (although a visit to the emergency room is still a good idea to remove all doubt).

Ouch!
Never attempt to drive a person who is having a heart attack to the hospital yourself. Only an ambulance is equipped with the space and the staff to perform CPR and check vital signs, or to deal with other unexpected emergencies and the heavy flow of traffic.

Strokes vs. Heart Attacks

The National Stroke Association defines a stroke as "a sudden disruption of the blood supply to a part of the brain, which, in turn, disrupts the body function controlled by that brain area." In short, you might call a stroke a "heart attack" of the brain.

There are technically four different types of strokes, but all of them have the same basic description: A blood clot or clogged artery prevents blood from continuing through the brain. The areas on the other side of this "medical dam" cannot receive the nutrient-rich blood they need to function. The result? Like a lawn that isn't watered in the heat of summer, the brain cells dry up and die.

Warning Signs of a Stroke

A stroke can occur as suddenly as a heart attack—when a person is walking down the street, driving a car, or sitting in a rowboat in the middle of a lake. With a stroke, however, the brain doesn't just shut down all at once. Depending on the location of the blockage, there may be any of several warning signs.

With a stroke, or TIA (Transient Ischemic Attack), the following symptoms last no more than 24 hours. More often than not, however, they signal the onset of a stroke:

➤ Sudden weakness or numbness of the face, arm, or leg on one side of the body only

➤ Sudden loss of speech, or trouble finding the right words

➤ Inability to comprehend what is being said

➤ Sudden dimness of bilateral (both eyes) vision, or loss of vision in one eye

➤ A sudden, very severe headache

➤ A sudden episode of dizziness or unsteadiness, or even a sudden fall

➤ Loss of bladder or bowel control

➤ Unconsciousness

➤ Very flushed face

Providing Emergency Treatment for a Stroke

As we've said over and over again, try to stay calm. Then call for help immediately. Before the emergency medical team arrives, follow these basic first aid steps:

1. Put the ill person in a semireclining position, if possible.

2. Loosen clothing around the neck and chest.

3. Check the victim's airways for blockage. Begin mouth-to-mouth resuscitation, if necessary (see Chapter 2).

4. Dab cool washcloths or cold compresses on the patient's neck and face.

5. If the person vomits, turn the head to the side and clean all vomit from his or her mouth.

6. Treat for shock, especially if the person is unconscious (see Chapter 2).

7. If the ill person has a muscle spasm or a seizure, do not attempt to restrain the person or force anything between his or her teeth. The victim might fall into a deep sleep after the seizure. This is quite common, so don't be alarmed.

Do You Know CPR?

CPR is short for cardiopulmonary resuscitation. If this procedure is begun immediately after someone has a heart attack, it can save his or her life. When performed properly, CPR can keep the blood circulating until help arrives. At that point, trained medical staff can use more sophisticated treatment en route to the hospital.

CPR is not difficult, but you need to be properly trained so that you can perform it without thinking (if you ever need to give someone CPR, you won't be in a position to stop and think about the steps). You can learn this skill in one or two sessions with a trained instructor. Almost every hospital offers CPR classes during the year, including special sessions on CPR for children, and you can also take CPR classes at your local YMCA.

Although CPR classes do cost some money, the fees aren't exorbitant. (And, after all, there is no price tag on life.) During the month of February—which has been dubbed "Heart Healthy Month"—many hospitals offer specials on CPR, sometimes giving classes for free, or for as little as $5. Check with your local hospital or YMCA for information about CPR classes.

Chapter 10

Extreme Temperatures: Too Much Sun or Snow

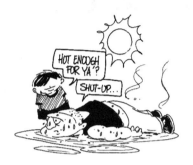

> **In This Chapter**
> ➤ Symptoms of too much sun and heat
> ➤ Symptoms of hypothermia
> ➤ Recognizing and treating frostbite

Especially in summer, the sun can cause sudden and serious problems, ones that a slathering of SPF 10 isn't going to help: heat prostration (also called heat exhaustion) and sunstroke. This chapter arms you with the first aid techniques for dealing with these conditions.

You'll also read about a different extreme: winter cold. Hypothermia (subnormal body temperature) can be just as deadly as heat prostration. It's especially common among people who exercise outdoors, people who cannot produce adequate body heat, and the elderly. Frostbite occurs as a result of extreme overexposure to cold. It can accompany hypothermia, or it can be a first aid emergency all by itself.

But first, the sun...

When the Sun Heats Up

Sun- and heat-related illnesses usually occur in the early summer, before people have adapted to the heat; and also later in the summer, during the dog days of July and August; during strenuous exercise (for example, running, cycling, or hiking) in the heat; and when an unexpected *heat wave* hits.

First Aids

A *heat wave* is more than just unusually high air temperature. For meteorologists to call a weather pattern an official heat wave, the high temperature must be combined with high humidity and a lack of wind. In other words, the air is close, hot, and stuffy, so you feel like you're trapped under a heavy wool blanket.

Although people sometimes use the terms *heat prostration, heat exhaustion,* and *sunstroke* interchangeably, in reality, only heat prostration and heat exhaustion are the same (and are distinct from sunstroke): a condition that occurs in an "overheated" body. Like an overheated car, the body's cooling mechanism slows down and fails to regulate body temperature quickly enough; a person begins to feel as if he or she has the flu and could display the following symptoms: confusion, chills, clammy skin, or flushed face. Heat prostration (or exhaustion) is rarely life threatening, but it must be treated. If you don't take care of an overheated body, unconsciousness, shock, and even death can result.

Sunstroke has symptoms similar to heat prostration, with one major difference: The body's cooling mechanism has completely stopped. It's not running slowly, it's stalled. Clearly, this element makes sunstroke and its consequent treatment more serious. It's important to recognize the subtle differences between heat prostration and sunstroke. Let's go over each condition now, covering everything from symptoms to first aid care.

Symptoms of Heat Prostration (Exhaustion)

If you notice someone suddenly experiencing any of the following symptoms, you can bet that he or she has fallen prey to heat prostration:

➤ Sudden high temperature, but under 104°F (a sudden temperature of only 100°F to 102°F can signal heat prostration in people over 65)

➤ Hot and flushed skin that might be clammy to the touch

➤ Muscle or stomach cramps

➤ Nausea and/or vomiting

➤ Headache

➤ Profuse sweating

➤ Rapid pulse

➤ Confusion

➤ Dizziness

➤ Chills

Treating Heat Prostration

Heat prostration (or exhaustion) is not usually a life-threatening condition, but it's still important to heed the following steps:

1. Get the ill person out of the sun.

2. Replace the body's lost fluids and salts by giving the victim lots of water, a sports drink, decaffeinated iced tea, or juice.

Ouch!

When suffering from heat exhaustion, you might be tempted to jump into the pool or the lake to cool off. Don't do it. If you go into the water with a case of heat exhaustion, you could end up with cramps; worse, you could pass out or have a seizure and drown.

3. Lower the person's body temperature with fans, cool towels, or sprays.

4. Keep the sufferer out of the sun for the next 12 to 24 hours.

A person who has suffered a bout of heat prostration needs to rest. The best bet is a full day of rest (or at least 12 hours), during which time he or she should catch up on lost fluids and give the body time to repair its systems. Once a person suffers heat prostration, he or she is more vulnerable to another occurrence of it (and to the more serious sunstroke)—rest is imperative.

Symptoms of Sunstroke

Sunstroke (also called heat stroke) is much more serious than heat prostration; keep in mind that if heat prostration is not treated promptly, it will escalate into sunstroke. Because the body's cooling mechanism shuts down altogether, sunstroke can be life threatening. Look for the following symptoms:

➤ Sudden, extremely high temperature (104°F or higher)

➤ Hot, flushed, very dry skin

➤ A total absence of sweating

➤ Rapid pulse

➤ Confusion

➤ Unconsciousness

➤ Convulsions

Treating Sunstroke

It's hard enough just to sit still and breathe when it's hot, sticky, and humid out and the sun is beating down unmercifully. Treating a person who's been overcome by these weather conditions is infinitely more difficult, both for you and the victim, but you must keep a cool head and follow these steps:

1. Call for help *immediately*—sunstroke is life threatening.

2. Immerse the ill person in a half-filled tub of cool water to lower body temperature. You can also sponge bathe the person with cool water. Make sure the water is cool, not teeth-chatteringly cold—comfort combined with effectiveness is key.

First Things First

If you can't get a sunstroke sufferer into a bathtub, wrap him or her in cool, water-soaked sheets and use a fan or the cool setting on a hair dryer to blow air on the body. You can also give the person a sponge bath with cool water from a pitcher or bucket.

3. Once the person's temperature is down, briskly towel him or her dry.

4. If the person is conscious and coherent, offer him or her plain water to drink while help is on its way. Do not give caffeinated drinks like soda.

Even if the person appears to have made a full recovery after you've administered first aid, make sure he or she gets medical attention.

The Other Extreme: Hypothermia

Just as too much heat and sun can cause illness, so can extreme cold. *Hypothermia* is the drastic loss of body heat that results from overexposure to the cold. A person suffering from hypothermia will have a sudden, abnormally low body temperature (below 95°), which will, in turn, slow down important physiological processes, such as breathing, swallowing, and blood circulation.

The symptoms of hypothermia occur suddenly and abruptly. They include:

➤ Fatigue, drowsiness, or a tremendous "need" to sleep

➤ Weakness

➤ Depressed, slow pulse

➤ Slow, barely noticeable breathing

➤ Low blood pressure

Hypothermia is rarely life threatening—if it's treated quickly enough. If you need to administer first aid for hypothermia, follow these steps:

1. Get the person indoors to warmth, but avoid radiators and fireplaces. These offer too extreme a change in temperature and can cause more harm.

2. Cover the person with a loose, warm blanket to prevent further loss of body heat. Getting under the blanket with them and sharing your natural body heat will also help warm up the victim.

3. If the person is conscious, appears lucid, and can swallow, you can offer him or her something warm and soothing to sip, but avoid alcohol.

4. If possible, observe the person for several hours. Cardiac arrest is not uncommon during hypothermia, and you'll need to be nearby to administer first aid, if necessary. (See Chapter 9 for details on heart attacks.)

The Nip of Winter Frostbite

Frostbite is the cold kissing cousin of hypothermia. It's quite common and almost never life threatening (although it can be serious enough for a person to lose part of a limb). It occurs most often in cold winter weather, especially when low temperatures are combined with a cold wind or wet conditions.

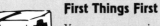

First Things First

You can recognize frostbite by its color. Frostbitten fingers or toes will first be bright red. Then they'll turn gray, then stark, icy white. (Darker skin will ultimately become an ashy gray color.)

You'll know you're suffering from frostbite when the affected body part starts to tingle or ache slightly and eventually becomes numb. As soon as you recognize its telltale symptoms, begin this treatment procedure:

1. Call for medical help immediately. The faster you get help, the less likely the victim will lose a limb.

2. Get the person in from the cold as quickly as possible and remove any wet or icy clothing.

3. Protect the frozen area of the body, "thawing" it out with lukewarm water. If water isn't available, use a warm, woolen blanket or natural body heat. (For example, you could put frostbitten fingers into the armpits, if you could stand it.) Do *not* use a hair dryer—that's too hot. Nor should you massage the frozen area. Rubbing it can actually cause tissue damage.

4. Within a half hour, feeling will return—and with it will come a lot of pain. The area will also become red and swollen. Although this might seem horrible, it's actually a good thing. It's a sign that blood is beginning to circulate in the area again.

5. Once the body part is thawed, keep it warm, dry, and clean until you see a physician—especially if feeling has not returned.

6. If blisters appear, apply an antibacterial ointment and a loose, sterile dressing.

Chapter 11

Ow! Sprains, Strains, Breaks, and Muscle Cramps

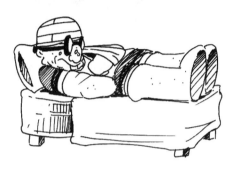

In This Chapter

➤ Treating cramps, strains, and sprains: Is there a difference?

➤ When a muscle cramp can signal something dangerous

➤ Sprains vs. breaks

A cramp can be a symptom of anything from intestinal gas to appendicitis—or even a heart attack. Likewise, a strain, which can result from being at the gym a half hour too long, can ultimately lead to inflamed muscles and painful pinched nerves.

Sprains and breaks, too, can be simple to handle or the start of something complicated. Obviously, a broken bone must be treated properly to ensure correct alignment as it heals. But a sprain is more subtle. It might just require an

Ace bandage and staying off your feet for a day or two; without the right treatment, however, a sprain can lead to swelling and pain and (eventually) chronic nerve, muscle, or bone damage and arthritis.

But never fear. By the time you finish reading this chapter, you'll know how to recognize these conditions, how to treat them, and how to prevent them from occurring in the first place.

Cramping Your Style: Muscle Cramps and Strains

A muscle cramp can be one of the fallouts of exercise, especially on hot days. Some of you might know firsthand what it feels like when a muscle in your arm or leg suddenly—and painfully—knots itself into a tight fist. Cramps can also occur when you move around in bed or even when you're simply taking a nap.

A muscle strain is more serious, especially when it affects the muscles in the back. A strain involves injury not only to muscles, but also to ligaments, tendons, or blood vessels surrounding a bone joint. The injured tissue is either pulled, stretched, wrenched, or torn during physical activity (like when you take a flying leap across the room during your first dance class in 30 years).

Treating Muscle Cramps

Muscle cramps are easy to fix and do not require emergency first aid. Treat them in this way:

1. Stretch out the muscle as soon as you feel a cramp.

2. Massage the knotted muscle with the heel of the hand for several minutes.

3. Follow the massage with a warm bath, a warm wet compress, or a heating pad to provide soothing heat. This should release the knot.

Muscle cramps commonly affect your calf or the heel of your foot while you're exercising or playing team sports. To stretch out the cramped leg (or foot), place the foot flat on the floor and bend the knee, making sure that the heel stays on the floor the whole time; see the following illustration. Hold this position while you massage the cramp.

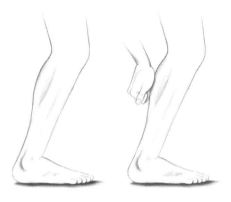

Stretch and massage cramped calves.

Treating Muscle Strains

You treat muscle strains by doing the exact opposite of what you would do for a cramp.

1. Do not stretch or massage the muscle; instead, keep it at rest. Ibuprofen can help ease the pain and reduce inflammation.

2. Elevate a strained arm or leg to prevent swelling.

3. Think *cold:* Place cold wet cloths or a cold compress on the muscle.

   The appropriate technique for "icing" an injury is to wrap ice in a clean cloth and alternately apply the ice to the injury for 20 minutes, remove the ice for 20 minutes, and reapply (with fresh ice) for 20 minutes. Repeat this cycle for the first full day. You need to keep the muscle cold for the first 24 hours to prevent the muscle fiber from swelling, which could touch a nerve and cause even more pain. (Put an ice pack on before you go to sleep, and try to relax. Obviously, you have to sleep and can't help but miss a few hours.)

4. After 24 hours, think *warm:* Use hot wet compresses to soothe the muscle. The warmth increases blood circulation and facilitates healing.

Warning Signs of Other Conditions

A muscle cramp can be a result of too much exercise or a sudden wrong move, but it can also signal too much stress—or worse. A recurring cramp could be a warning sign of a serious disease. Check with your physician.

When your neck and shoulders cramp up, it's a good idea to stop what you're doing, roll your head from side to side, and shrug your shoulders. Relaxation exercises and meditation can also help this side effect of stress.

When your stomach cramps, it could be a sign of gastric distress or even appendicitis. And as your mother used to warn you, stomach cramps in the water can be serious. You won't necessarily get a stomach cramp from going swimming after a meal, but if you do, you could lose control and drown.

Strains, too, can lead to more serious situations. A strained back can leave you incapacitated for days—or weeks. Sometimes simple strains are combined with broken bones. And a severe strain might signal internal bleeding and swelling. If a strain doesn't go away after you follow the basic first aid treatment, see a physician.

Sprains and Breaks

Whether it happens to a child or an adult, a sprain or break (also called a fracture) can be serious. Depending on its location, a broken bone can be life threatening. It can lead to shock, a weak pulse, or breathing difficulties. And at the very least, a sprain or break hurts—a lot.

The steps you take to treat a sprain or break while you're waiting to get professional care can make the difference in whether a break heals correctly and in proper alignment.

The Differences Between Sprains and Breaks

How different are sprains and breaks? Not much. A sprain is a strain taken to the max. A sprain is kind of like a strain at the bone itself; the muscle fibers, connective tissues, or ligaments of a joint have been stretched to their limits or wrenched completely out of whack.

As you might guess, a break goes one step further: The bone actually breaks. In fact, a break doesn't have to occur only at muscle junctures, such as the elbow or ankle. Bones can break anywhere along their mass, from lower arms to upper thighs, from buttocks and hips to collarbones.

Only with an x-ray can you definitively tell whether a bone is broken. Because sprains and breaks can look similar, you should treat every sprain as if it were a break, and you should have it x-rayed. It's better to be safe than sorry.

Signs of bone injury or joint sprain include:

➤ Feeling or hearing an actual "snap"

➤ Bluish discoloration or bruising over the injured bone or joint

➤ Abnormal position of a limb

➤ Inability to move a limb on one's own

➤ Excessive pain at injury site

➤ Swelling, numbness, and tingling near injured bone or joint

Treating Sprains and Breaks

There are four basic rules when it comes to first aid for bones:

➤ Bandage the sprain or break to keep injured arms, legs, shoulders, feet, and hands immobile. Chapter 2 contains step-by-step instructions for bandaging different parts of the body.

➤ Get the injured person to an emergency treatment location as soon as possible.

➤ Keep the injured person immobile to prevent further injury and excessive pain.

➤ While you're waiting, watch the person's vital signs and check those ABCs (Airways clear, Breathing regular, Circulation steady). You do not want the injured person to go into shock (see Chapter 2).

Ouch!
Never give a person with a broken bone anything to eat or drink or any medication to swallow. Depending on the vicinity of the broken bone, it can block a blood vessel, further damage the gut, lungs, or other organs, or create breathing problems.

Chapter 12

(Don't) Choose Your Poison

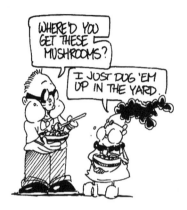

In This Chapter

➤ Common poisons in the home: cleaning products, food, pesticides, and drugs

➤ Carbon monoxide: the invisible poison

➤ Recognizing and dealing with food poisoning

Poison, poison everywhere. Unfortunately, it comes in many forms that you might accidentally drink, inhale, apply, or eat—you should always be careful. Many poisons are commonly found in the home, so you should make sure they're safely locked away, out of children's reach.

Poisoning happens much less in real life than it does on television or in best-selling mystery novels, but it can happen. When it does, you need to know how to perform first aid care.

Always Contact the Poison Control Center

Put down this book immediately (mark your place, of course) and find your telephone book. Look up the number of your local poison control center and record it on your list of emergency phone numbers, tape it in your first aid kit, post it on your refrigerator door, and keep it in your glove compartment.

If you suspect someone is suffering from a poison—from food, household detergents, carbon monoxide, or drugs, for example—call that poison control center number first, even before you call an emergency medical team.

Why?

When seconds count, you need to know exactly what to do, and that varies depending on what caused the poisoning. Some poisons need to be expelled from the body through induced vomiting. Others should never be thrown up because they'll cause as much or more damage on the way back up as they did on the way down. The poison control center can give you step-by-step instructions for what to do while you're waiting on an ambulance or stuck in traffic driving to the emergency ward. If possible, be prepared to answer the following questions:

➤ What kind of poison was ingested?

➤ How much and how long ago?

➤ How old is the victim?

➤ What are the symptoms? Has he or she vomited?

➤ Have you given him or her anything to drink? If yes, what?

The more you can tell the poison control center, the more its specialists can help you.

When to Induce Vomiting

It sounds logical. To get rid of poison that's been swallowed, the best thing is vomit it up, right? Wrong. In most cases, vomiting is the ideal antidote. But there are times when it's best to keep the poison down and wait for emergency medical help.

First Things First
If you don't know what the victim has ingested, do *not* induce vomiting. It's far better to be safe than to possibly cause more harm.

Only your local poison control center can tell you for sure whether it's good to vomit. If you cannot reach your local poison control center, you'll have to make a judgment call. Do *not* induce vomiting under any of the following conditions:

➤ Someone has swallowed a cleaning product containing acids or alkalis. These substances can severely burn throat tissue as the victim throws up.

➤ Someone has swallowed a petroleum-based product. These types of cleaners exude fumes that can cause pneumonia if inhaled. When the poisoned person vomits, these fumes can be inhaled—by both you and the victim.

➤ The victim is groggy or confused.

➤ The victim is too young to understand and follow directions (such as a baby under two years old).

➤ You are in doubt. The person's age, the delay time, and the amount ingested all factor into the equation.

How to Induce Vomiting

We can't repeat it enough: Call the poison control center immediately when someone ingests a poison. If the authorities at the poison control center give you the go-ahead to induce vomiting and eliminate the ingested poison, follow these important steps:

1. Give an adult patient two tablespoons of syrup of ipecac; give a child patient one tablespoon; give a baby (less than 12 months old) two teaspoons.

2. Follow the syrup with four or five glasses of water.

3. Make sure the person's head is lowered to prevent choking. Inside, an adult or child can lie across a bed with his head off the side; outside, he can kneel with his head bent. If a baby swallows poison, hold the baby on your lap with the head down, supporting the head on your lap with your hand.

4. Try to have the ill person vomit into a bowl so that you can take it along to the emergency ward with the victim for analysis.

5. If the patient does not vomit, try to induce vomiting again in 20 minutes.

6. If the ill person still does not vomit, don't give him or her any more syrup. Instead, insert your finger in his or her throat to stimulate vomiting via the gagging reflex.

7. After the person vomits, mix one ounce of activated charcoal (if available) in water and have the person sip it. This calms the stomach and acts as a temporary neutralizing antidote.

8. Keep the poisoned person warm.

9. Keep the person calm. He or she might become panicked. Soothe as best you can. As a last resort,

restrain the person using a belt, but only if the person's agitation is so great that it could cause injury.

10. Mind your ABCs of first aid: Make sure that Airways are clear, Breathing is fairly normal, and Circulation (via pulse) is okay (see Chapter 1).

If necessary, treat for shock or resuscitate the victim (see Chapter 2). Also, if the ill person begins to have a convulsion, do not try to restrain him or her, and do not force anything between the teeth.

When to Avoid Vomiting

Preventing a person from vomiting can be as difficult as inducing him or her to vomit, especially if the person has ingested something particularly nauseating and painful. If you're treating a person who has ingested a poison for which induced vomiting is not advised, follow these steps:

First Things First

If vomiting seems inevitable, turn the person's head to the side so that the airways aren't blocked. Try to get him or her to swallow and take deep breaths between vomiting.

1. Call 911 and get medical help as fast as you can.

2. Place the person on his or her back. This will keep the reflex action subdued.

3. Keep the person's head down, on a pillow.

4. Keep the person calm and comfortable until help arrives.

Knowing What to Avoid

Why would anyone eat rhubarb leaves or azalea bushes? Good question—unless you happen to be two years old. Curiosity killed the cat, and it has often harmed a child. Pretty berries, leaves, and flowers are easy prey for the young, curious mind. Of course, adults might also inadvertently eat poisonous plants—if, for example, someone were cooking with rhubarb or eggplant for the first time and didn't know that their leaves were poisonous.

Chemicals are another matter altogether. Sometimes children drink household poisons because the colors on the container are "pretty." (Do you need a better reason to childproof your home?) And there have also been cases in which adults have swallowed household poisons as a means of attempting suicide.

Ouch!

Even bad-tasting, foul-smelling plants, chemicals, and medications won't stop fearless young "explorers." Many children will sample a poison even as they're turning up their noses. So keep all poisons in childproof cabinets or containers and keep them out of sight.

To prevent or deal with any of these scenarios, you should be aware of the types of poisons lurking in and around your home. Poisonous plants (or plant parts) include: apple seeds, azalea bushes, castor bean seeds, iris flowers, jonquil bulbs, lilies-of-the-valley, pointsettia leaves, potato greens, rhododendron bushes, daffodil bulbs, eggplant leaves, holly berries, mistletoe berries, narcissus bulbs, philodendron leaves, rhubarb leaves, sweet pea seeds, and tomato foliage. You should also childproof your home, keeping household cleaning agents, deodorants, detergents, laundry bleaches, prescription and over-the-counter medications, and fuels (such as kerosene) away from curious hands. For a more complete listing of poisonous substances, call your local poison control center.

Drug Overdoses: Accidents Waiting to Happen to Children

Many drug overdoses involve children who go exploring in the family medicine cabinet. When left unsupervised, children can get into pills and medications that can be harmful to their health. Ninety percent of all reported drug poisonings occur in children under five years old.

Accidental drug overdoses aren't limited to children. An adult might not realize, for example, that she is allergic to a certain medication. Or she might not know what a lethal combination two different types of medication can be. Or maybe she just forgets that she already took her prescribed dosage and she takes it again. Of course, drug overdoses can also be deliberate—those are the saddest cases of all.

The best first aid treatment for accidental or deliberate drug overdose is *prevention*. Follow these safety guidelines:

➤ Childproof all cabinets you keep medicine in, and keep safety caps on all pill bottles.

➤ Read all labels on medications before taking them, especially the warning labels pertaining to complications that result from medicine combinations.

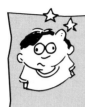

Ouch!

Aspirin is the drug most commonly involved in accidental poisonings of children. One bottle of baby aspirin containing 50 pills can kill a child!

➤ Keep medicines (even vitamins) away from food. They belong in the medicine cabinet, not the spice drawer.

➤ From time to time, give your children the medicine "rap": Pills are not candy. Medicine is not good to eat. Pills can be downright dangerous.

Use these poison symbols to label dangerous substances.

Poisons That You Don't Eat or Drink

Poison can take many forms. In addition to being swallowed, it can be absorbed through the skin or inhaled. The air you breathe can hold dangerous toxins. And if some harsh, chemical household products (such as drain cleaners and dishwasher powder) come into contact with your skin, they can cause burns or poisonous reactions—it can be almost as bad as if you'd swallowed them.

How Sweet It Isn't: Breathing in Carbon Monoxide

The most common poisonous gas in the home is carbon monoxide, the odorless, invisible gas that is emitted by cars and some heating systems. Although it's always present, carbon monoxide becomes dangerous only when it reaches certain levels and when it's trapped in an enclosed space.

Symptoms of carbon monoxide poisoning include the following:

➤ Flushed skin

➤ Bright, cherry-red lips

➤ Dizziness

➤ Weakness

➤ Headache

These symptoms ultimately lead to memory loss, confusion, and unconsciousness.

Ouch!
Never leave your car running in the garage with the garage doors closed. Although you might not smell the noxious fumes, they can cause you to lose consciousness quickly—and die within a few hours.

Follow these first aid steps immediately to help someone overcome by carbon monoxide or some other poisonous gas:

1. If in a garage, turn off the engine and open the doors of the car and the garage.

2. Loosen his or her clothing.

3. Call for emergency medical help.

4. Keep the ill person on the ground. Tip the head to the side to ensure clear airways in case he or she vomits.

5. Begin mouth-to-mouth resuscitation, if necessary, while you wait for help to arrive.

Chemical and Gas Fumes First Aid Rescue

It can come out of nowhere: a gas burner's pilot light that's left on, a broken heater in the home, a malfunction in your RV's air system, an exterminator's strong fumes, or wet paint left to dry in an unventilated space. When these types of chemical and gas fumes are inhaled or absorbed into the skin, they can be as dangerous as carbon monoxide. And as with carbon monoxide poisoning, the first order of (first aid) business is to get anyone who is affected by such fumes out into the fresh air as soon as possible. To rescue someone in a fume-filled room, follow these steps:

1. Call for help immediately, especially if you're alone. Just in case you, too, are overcome, it's important to know that someone is on the way to rescue you.

2. Before you enter the room, take several deep breaths of fresh air. Try to hold your breath as long as you can when you rush into the room.

3. If the victim is in an area that cannot be ventilated before you enter (an underground tank, for example), it's best to wait for professional help to arrive—you don't want to end up a "dead" hero. And never enter a room or corridor alone if the victim is not near the exit. Again, you might not get out alive.

4. If there is someone else who can help you with the rescue attempt, you can tie a rope around your waist

and give the loose end of the rope to the other person (or vice versa) before you enter the room. That way, you can use the rope as a lifeline if you're overcome by the fumes in the room.

5. If the fumes are visible and circling near the floor, keep your head high. If the fumes appear to be closer to the ceiling, crouch down and walk or crawl underneath them.

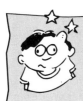

Ouch!

It might seem obvious, but we'll say it anyway: Fumes can be explosive. *Never light a match in a fume-filled room.*

6. Grasp the overcome person and get him or her out of the room as fast as you can.

7. Once you're in the fresh air, check the victim's breathing. If he or she is not breathing, immediately proceed with mouth-to-mouth resuscitation (see Chapter 2), or if you're trained, begin CPR.

   If the victim seems to be clear-headed, awake, and breathing fine, have him lie on his back. Elevate his legs by placing a pillow under the lower legs; this keeps blood circulating and ensures that the brain gets plenty of oxygen.

   If the victim is having trouble breathing, lay him on his back with his head resting on an elevated pillow while you wait for help. (If he is overcome by smoke, see Chapter 7.)

   If the victim is unconscious, place a pillow under his head and position him on his side to keep airways clear in case vomiting occurs (see the illustration below).

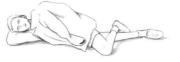

Position an unconscious victim on his side and bend the top knee so that he won't roll over.

8. Check the victim's skin and eyes for possible contamination. If the eyes are very irritated or burned, it's possible that they've come in contact with chemical fumes. Flush the eyes immediately with cool water. (Chapter 8 covers first aid treatment for eye injuries.)

9. If the skin is burned from fumes or from contact with chemicals, pour cool water on the wound and try to flush out the poison. (Chapter 3 covers first aid treatment for skin irritations.)

Even if the victim seems fine once you've rescued him or her, it's a good idea to make a doctor's appointment within the next few days. Inhalation of poisonous fumes can cause side effects such as nerve damage, respiratory problems, memory loss, and muscle aches, some of which don't appear right away.

Food Poisoning

We've all read reports about undercooked chicken and pork, mayonnaise and eggs left out in the sun too long, and seafood that's gone from not fresh to bad. What changes these foods from delicious delights to dangerous disasters? Bacteria, that's what.

When food is left out in the sun, when meats are not thoroughly cooked, or when fish spoils, these foods become breeding grounds for all kinds of organisms, from bacteria to parasites. In the following sections, we cover the three most common types of bacteria that you can ingest by eating undercooked or spoiled food.

Staphylococcus

It might sound like a mouthful—and it is. The most common type of food poisoning is named from the bacteria that contaminates foods such as mayonnaise left out in the sun, cream or custards that are not fresh, soured milk, and unrefrigerated meats. Those foods provide prime growing ground for the staphylococcus bacteria.

Symptoms of this type of bacterial poisoning will occur almost immediately or within only a few hours. They include nausea and vomiting, diarrhea, stomach pain, and weakness.

The best treatment for staphylococcal poisoning is patience. The symptoms will usually clear up (and out) within a few hours. During that time, make sure the ill person is comfortable and near a bathroom. Do not give him or her any pills or medication, but give water if it's requested.

Salmonella

Despite its name, salmonella doesn't just occur in salmon. It, too, is a bacteria—a more serious cousin of staphylococcus. Salmonella poisoning occurs in contaminated foods, cooked and raw. It's also linked to poor sanitary conditions. (In other words, avoid food stores swarming with insects, heat, and unsanitary food handlers.)

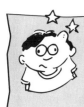

Ouch!
Salmonella bacteria is most prevalent in undercooked and improperly cleaned or stored poultry, pork, beef, and eggs.

Symptoms of salmonella poisoning usually surface about eight hours after a person eats the bad food. The symptoms are very similar to those of staphylococcal poisoning, but they are much more severe.

If you think someone might have salmonella poisoning, seek medical help immediately. Then make the person as comfortable as possible. Give him or her only water, if requested.

First Things First
Avoid the possibility of salmonella poisoning by washing your hands before and after handling raw meats, poultry, and eggs; don't forget to wash your countertops, cutting boards, and knives, too. Always store these foods in the refrigerator.

Botulinum

The most devious food poisoning, botulism, is also the most deadly. It's an illness caused by the botulinum bacteria. Symptoms usually don't appear until two days after ingestion—it can sometimes be difficult to trace back to the contaminated food. Botulism is caused by contamination of canned goods; the botulinum bacteria thrives on improperly packaged food and food that is used after it has "turned bad." New studies also reveal that botulism can occur in gourmet, hand-flavored bottled oils, in which whole slivers of peppers or herbs are placed in a glass bottle along with the cooking oil.

Botulinum bacteria produces symptoms all its own:

➤ Blurriness or dim vision

➤ Double vision

➤ Heavy eyelids

➤ Difficulty breathing

➤ Severe fatigue

➤ Inability to swallow

➤ Garbled speech

First Things First
How can you tell if the food in a can might have been contaminated? If a can is battered, swollen at the top or bottom, sold after the "best used by" date, or exudes a strong odor when it's opened, the food's probably bad. When in doubt, throw it out.

If any of these symptoms occur, seek medical assistance immediately. Try to remember what the ill person ate over the past two days and find the culprit. Pinpointing the food can help the emergency team provide the correct treatment. If the ill person cannot remember what she consumed or if she is too sick to talk, try to retrace her steps by checking her appointment book, calling her office, and looking in her garbage can.

Chapter 13

Sticks and Stones: Splinters and Puncture Wounds

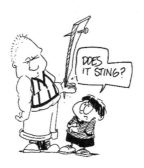

DOES IT STING?

In This Chapter

➤ How to take out a splinter

➤ Recognizing the signs of infection

➤ What to do when impaled objects cannot be removed

Splinters and puncture wounds are very similar: A foreign object punctures or impales the skin. The difference between the two is a matter of degree. Splinters are relatively minor, and you can usually handle their removal without outside help. Puncture wounds, on the other hand, penetrate farther below the skin, possibly damaging blood vessels, muscles, and nerves. For those, you'll always need emergency help.

A Splinter Is a Splinter Is a Splinter...

Who hasn't had a splinter at one time or another? A tiny sliver of glass, a minuscule piece of wood, a slender slice of plastic or metal—it slides right under the skin and lodges itself there, causing you pain. These splinters might hurt, but if they are removed properly, you won't suffer any infection. To take out a splinter, follow these step-by-step instructions:

1. Place the instrument you'll be using to remove the splinter nearby. The instrument is usually a plain sewing needle or tweezers, or both.

2. Wash your hands thoroughly with soap and water, and wash the splinter site to make conditions as sterile as possible.

3. Sterilize the sewing needle and tweezers you will use to take out the splinter by either dropping them in boiling water for 10 minutes or heating them over the flame of a match or lighter. (Wipe off any black carbon deposits with a sterile gauze pad.)

First Things First

Clear glass splinters, by their very nature, are difficult to see, especially if the slivers are tiny. To ensure that you've gotten the entire splinter out, look through a magnifying glass under a bright light.

4. Using the sewing needle or tweezers, gently and carefully brush the skin and its tiny hairs from the splinter area, layer by layer.

5. When enough of the splinter is exposed to be able to grab it, use your tweezers and pull it out. If the

splinter is small, continue to use the sewing needle, working out the splinter from the skin.

6. Brush the skin with the sewing needle a little more to make sure you've gotten all of the splinter. Think of the needle as a little broom, pushing away the skin tissue surrounding the point of insertion. This is especially important when a sliver of glass is the culprit.

7. Wash the wound area with water, whether it's bleeding or not. Apply an antibacterial ointment.

8. Cover the clean wound site with a Band-Aid or gauze pad and tape.

Puncture Wounds

A puncture wound leaves a small hole on the surface of the skin, but below the surface the foreign object is deeply embedded. The wound spreads under the skin, causing bleeding and tissue damage.

Most puncture wounds are caused by objects bigger than splinters. Arrows, large shards of metal and glass, nails, and even sharp sticks of wood can puncture the skin and damage underlying tissue.

The Hidden Problems with Punctures

Any puncture wound is prone to infection because of the depth of the foreign object's invasion. Particularly vulnerable are those punctures in which a foreign object:

➤ Goes through clothing, taking particles of cloth with it as it enters the skin

➤ Breaks up into smaller pieces as it becomes embedded under the skin

➤ Is extremely dirty, such as a rusty nail

➤ Enters the body through the foot—it can get pushed in farther as a person tries to limp toward help

Signs of infection include redness at the puncture site, swelling (especially if blood vessels have been damaged), tenderness near the wound, and localized pain. You're not totally out of the woods just because these signs do not appear the day of the injury. Another sign of infection, oozing pus, can appear days after the accident.

If after a few days the wound scabs over, the redness disappears, and swelling at the site of impact goes down, you can usually say that the danger of infection is gone. But if pus continues (or starts) to drain from the site and the redness persists, it could very well mean that infection has set in—or that the foreign object left a souvenir. (This is particularly dangerous because even very small foreign objects, which are deeply embedded in the skin, can cause infection and blood poisoning.) At this point, it's important for you to take the victim to a physician, a medicenter, or the emergency room for better treatment. An antibiotic might have to be prescribed to fight the infection.

First Aids

Tetanus is an infectious, sometimes fatal disease caused by a bacterium that invades the body through wounds. Its symptoms include violent spasms and paralysis of the neck and jaw. For this reason, the disease is often called "lockjaw."

Sometimes when a puncture wound occurs, the object enters the body tissue, but does not remain embedded in it. This is what happens when a person steps on a rusty nail hammered into a piece of wood or leans against an immobile sharp edge. When it comes to rusty nails and shards of dirty glass, it doesn't matter whether an object is embedded. Don't wait. Go to your physician or emergency room as soon as possible. You can clean the wound and apply antiseptic by yourself first. A rusty nail could cause a bad infection or tetanus, and the victim might need a tetanus shot. If the victim hasn't had a tetanus shot within the past 10 years, he or she will need a booster. Tetanus bacteria thrives in dark, deep places with little air—like puncture wounds.

Treating a Puncture Wound

The first rule to remember: Do not try to remove an object embedded in a puncture wound by yourself. Any movement can cause more tissue damage or more bleeding. Call for emergency help and keep the puncture site immobile using these steps:

1. Gently clean the wound with soap and water, and then cover the wound with a loose gauze pad and adhesive tape.

2. Poke a hole in the bottom of a paper cup wide enough to slip over the exposed end of the foreign object.

3. Gently tape the cup to the body, so that it doesn't slip. Make a "fence" of cardboard or newspaper if you don't have a cup. See the following figure.

4. If the puncture wound is on the arm, further immobilize the wound by keeping the arm tight against the torso. Do this by winding a scarf or belt around both the arm (farther down from the wound) and lower torso.

   If the puncture wound is on the leg, wind the cloth or belt around both legs, adding a sturdy piece of wood to the back of the legs for extra insurance.

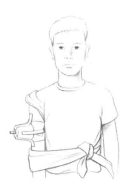

Immobilize a puncture wound to prevent more damage.

Dealing with Bleeding

As with any bleeding wound, applying direct pressure stops the flow of blood. (See Chapter 2 for more information on bleeding.) If the injured person is bleeding profusely, do not immobilize the wound immediately. Before you take any other action, stop the bleeding using these steps:

1. Cut any clothing away from the wound.

2. Wash your hands thoroughly to avoid further infection to the wound.

3. Put a sterile gauze pad *around* the embedded object, but not directly on it. If the object is protruding, place the gauze pad on the skin and encircle the site of penetration.

4. Remember the earlier instructions for treating puncture wounds. Cut a hole in the bottom of a paper cup and slide it over any protruding objects. Secure the cup to the body. This will keep infection at bay until you can get help.

5. Press firmly on the gauze pad surrounding the cup.

6. Keep the wound elevated above heart level, if possible, to lessen the blood flow to the site.

Glossary of First Aid

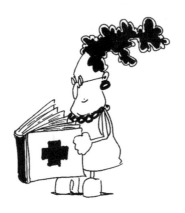

ABCs of first aid   Remembering these ABCs in the correct order will help you save a life: Make sure that **A**irways are open, **B**reathing is restored, and **C**irculation is maintained.

Ace bandage   An elastic strip of material, secured with hooks, that wraps around a sprained limb to keep the injury secure.

acute asthma   Associated with shortness of breath accompanied by wheezing. During an attack, the bronchial tubes constrict, impairing the flow of air into the lungs.

airway bag   An apparatus that provides a protective barrier between you and the victim and facilitates "breathing" into the victim's lungs during mouth-to-mouth resuscitation.

anaphylactic reaction   An allergic reaction, usually to bee stings, in which the throat swells up so much that a person eventually won't be able to breathe. A prescription antihistamine and epinephrine must be administered immediately to neutralize the reaction.

antihistamine   An over-the-counter pill, such as Benadryl, that stops the sneezing and sniffling of an allergy attack.

cardiac arrest   A condition in which the heart suddenly stops beating.

Cardiopulmonary Resuscitation (CPR)   A special rhythmic resuscitation technique used when the heart stops beating. Training is required to do CPR correctly.

concussion   A bang on the head. Although an outside wound can sometimes show, most of the damage is done inside, where the brain hits the skull. Most concussions are minor, clearing up after a few days of rest.

Emergency Medical Technician (EMT)   A trained professional who comes in a fully supplied ambulance when you call for help.

frostbite   A condition in which parts of the body "freeze" and are left without circulation. Frostbite is characterized by redness, then gray-colored skin, which eventually turns a bright, icy color (the signal of tissue damage).

heat prostration   A condition that occurs from too much sun and dehydration. Symptoms include a temperature less than 104°F and profuse sweating. (In the elderly, heat prostration occurs when the body temperature reaches 100°F to 102°F.)

Heimlich Maneuver   A technique used to dislodge whatever is causing a person to choke. Named after its inventor, U.S. surgeon Henry J. Heimlich, this maneuver literally pushes out the food or object that is causing breathing problems.

hemorrhage   Excessive bleeding.

hyperventilation   A condition of rapid overbreathing that occurs in acute anxiety attacks. Symptoms of the anxiety attack include numbness in the hands, feet, and mouth, a tingling sensation in the fingers and toes, an overwhelming feeling of panic, and an inability to catch one's breath.

ice compress   A cloth wrapped over ice or a chemically cold, flexible packet that is put on bumps, bruises, strains, and sprains to reduce swelling.

immobilize   To keep an injured person completely still (especially important when a head or back injury is suspected). Immobilization can be achieved by using pillows as a brace and belts as straps.

Medic Alert bracelet   A bracelet or necklace that contains vital health information about the person wearing it: allergies, diabetes, or epilepsy. It also gives a phone number that you can call to receive a more complete medical history. Always look for Medic Alert bracelets when a victim is unconscious.

mouth-to-mouth resuscitation   Used to resuscitate someone who has stopped breathing, this technique involves exhaling directly into the victim's mouth.

pulse   The rhythmic swelling and shrinking of the arteries as the blood moves through them. Take the pulse at the inner wrist, at the side of the neck, and at the temple.

shock   A condition in which the body's chemistry suddenly, immediately, and rapidly goes out of whack. Symptoms include erratic breathing, clammy and pale skin, chills and nausea, weakness, and unconsciousness.

sling   A triangular brace used to keep broken arms immobile and secured.

spiral technique   A bandaging technique used to wrap knees and upper legs securely.

splint   A device used to support and immobilize broken bones, fractures, sprains, and painful joints. A splint is any hard, straight object that is bandaged to the limb in question.

stroke   A sudden disruption of the blood supply to a part of the brain, which, in turn, disrupts the body function controlled by that brain area (definition from The National Stroke Association).

syrup of ipecac   A liquid that induces vomiting.

tetanus   An infection, also known as "lockjaw," that literally paralyzes its victims.

tourniquet   A device used when bleeding is so heavy that finger pressure doesn't stop it. A tourniquet can be anything from a belt to a shirt that is tied tightly a few inches above the cut to stop blood flow.

universal safety guidelines   New official rules and regulations that hospital staff, physicians, and health care professionals must follow in order to prevent transmission of disease or highly infectious viruses, such as HIV. An example of a universal safety guideline is always wearing latex gloves when treating a patient.

Emergency Medical Info

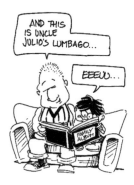

Use this chart to keep track of your family's medical history and important or emergency telephone numbers.

Telephone Numbers

Poison Control Center _____

Police _____

Fire Dept _____

Ambulance _____

Nearest Drug Store _____

24-hour Drug Store _____

Gas Company _____

Electric Company _____

Dentist _____

24-hour Taxi _____

Other _____

Family Medical Chart

Family Member	Allergies	Medical Problems	Medications	Date of Last Tetanus Shot	Phone Number at Work or School

Doctor	For Which Family Member(s)?	Address	Phone Number

In Case of Emergency Contact

Neighbor	Address	Phone Number

Index

U – V

W–X–Y–Z

About the Authors

Stephen J. Rosenberg, M.D., is a board-certified neurologist who has had a thriving practice in Orlando, Florida, for more than 30 years. Dr. Rosenberg graduated *cum laude* from Princeton University, and he went on to graduate from the University of Pennsylvania School of Medicine. He is an expert in geriatric emergencies and is currently the Associate Medical Director of the Brain Injury Rehabilitation Center at Orlando Regional Health Services. Dr. Rosenberg is also a Clinical Associate Professor of Medicine at the University of Florida School of Medicine, and an Attending Physician and member of the Medical Teaching Staff at the Orlando Regional Medical Center. He is a Fellow of the American Academy of Neurology and has received the Attending Physician of the Year Award, given by the Medical Teaching Service at the Orlando Regional Medical Center. He has also received a Certificate of Appreciation for services to the Veterans Administration at the Orlando Outpatient Clinic, and he is on the Board of the National Multiple Sclerosis Society.

Karla Dougherty is the author of 25 nonfiction books, many of them on medical topics. She is a member of the Author's Guild and the American Medical Writers Association. Karla lives in Montclair, New Jersey.